G000125318

PRAYER JOURNEY
INTO PARENTHOOD

Claire Daniel

The Bible Reading Fellowship
15 The Chambers, Vineyard
Abingdon OX14 3FE
brf.org.uk

The Bible Reading Fellowship (BRF) is a Registered Charity (233280)

ISBN 978 0 85746 479 8
First published 2016
10 9 8 7 6 5 4 3 2 1 0
All rights reserved

Text © Claire Daniel 2016
The author asserts the moral right to be identified as the author of this work

Cover images: © Thinkstock

Acknowledgements

Unless otherwise stated, scripture quotations are taken from The Holy Bible, New International Version (Anglicised edition) copyright © 1979, 1984, 2011 by Biblica. Used by permission of Hodder & Stoughton Publishers, an Hachette UK company. All rights reserved. 'NIV' is a registered trademark of Biblica. UK trademark number 1448790.

Every effort has been made to trace and contact copyright owners for material used in this resource. We apologise for any inadvertent omissions or errors, and would ask those concerned to contact us so that full acknowledgement can be made in the future.

A catalogue record for this book is available from the British Library

Printed and bound by Gutenberg Press Ltd.

PRAYER JOURNEY
INTO PARENTHOOD

Claire Daniel

BRF

Dedicated to my boys—Gary, Ewan and Benjamin

My fellow travellers on the journey
through pregnancy and into parenthood.
The adventure continues!

Acknowledgements

Thank you, firstly, to all those at BRF involved at every stage of developing my thoughts and reflections into this 'prayer journey into parenthood'. Special thanks to Naomi Starkey and Mike Parsons for your support and encouragement.

Mum and Charles and Chris and Graham, for your endless love, encouragement, support and prayers. Thank you for giving us your time, for entertaining grandchildren and for every little and huge thing you do to support us in our parenting journey.

My APC prayer ladies, Hannah, Vicky and Liz: thank you for listening and for praying me through the steps on the road to publication. Thanks to all our APC friends who have upheld us in prayer and walked with us on this journey.

To Paul and Carolyn, thank you for the peaceful writing haven you offered in our time of transition. Thanks to you and all at ST.P and ST.Ps who have welcomed us so warmly into our Water Orton church family.

Sam and Spud, your friendship means so much and we so appreciate your encouragement and wisdom as we share life and our journey through parenthood. Special thanks to Sam and Hannah J for your reassurance: you are amazing mums and I am hugely blessed to have your friendship.

My heartfelt thanks to Dr Harrison and Dr Flenley for refusing to give up until we found the cause of our infertility and for helping us on the path to diagnosis, on the road to pregnancy and over every medical bump in the road.

Dad and Grandpa Hooley, thank you for always supporting my endeavours. I am so glad that you were part of the beginning of our journey into parenthood. You were always so very proud of your children and grandchildren. I know you would have agreed that our two boys are one of my greatest achievements and would have been delighted to see this book published.

Gary, for being my rock, my constant support and companion on the journey into parenthood. Thank you for always encouraging me, working out this parenting lark together and sharing the load. My boys, Ewan and Benjamin, you amaze me daily and being your Mummy has taught me more than I can put into words.

Thank you, Lord, that you are my source of incredible strength and hope. Thank you that you have entrusted me once more with the incredible challenge and privilege of giving birth to a baby boy and a book, providing the inspiration and grace I needed to write, alongside my parenting journey.

------ *Contents* ------

Section One PREGNANCY PRAYER JOURNEY

Section Two PARENTHOOD PRAYER JOURNEY

Foreword

Last week I went to my godson's confirmation service. It took place within the ancient, cool walls of Salisbury's stunning cathedral. Right at the heart of the building, in contrast to its traditional surroundings, sits a contemporary font, which was installed in 2008. Unusually, the waters in this font have been designed to sit perfectly still across the water's surface, with mini fountains flowing from each of its four corners.

As I walked around the beautiful structure, my very pregnant body reflected back at me in the glasslike water, I was struck once again by the promise of Isaiah 43:2, inscribed around the font's edge: 'When you pass through the waters, I will be with you; and when you pass through the rivers, they will not sweep over you' (NIV).

When Claire asked me to write a foreword for this book, she was unaware that I was pregnant with our third child. Once again I am navigating the sometimes literally sick-making and at other times heart-bustingly joyful open waters of pregnancy, with childbirth and the excitement of meeting our newest family member just weeks away.

There's nothing quite like pregnancy to put your faith to the test. A life-changing, history-altering event takes place within your own body for a whole nine months—yet it is entirely outside your control and entirely unseen (apart from the bump and the selection of strange pregnancy symptoms that, admittedly, do tend to give the game away).

Then there's the birth—transformative, all-encompassing, mind-blowing—which takes place on a day, sometimes in a place and often in a way almost entirely outside your control.

Beyond this lie the wonderful days of starting to get to know the unique person with whom God has gifted you, who you have carried faithfully for months. And yet, mixed in with the wonder and praise for this miracle come the sleepless nights, anxiety and sometimes even depression.

The presence of God, real communication with him through prayer and the power of his Spirit at work in our everyday lives are needed like never before.

It's in your quest for a life-giving, sustaining relationship with Jesus, through this season of your life, that this book will help you. Claire has thoughtfully drawn together relevant Bible verses and prayers, alongside her own honest, real and thoughtful reflections on becoming a mum of two. Becoming a parent was not an easy journey for Claire and her husband, and she has graciously and sensitively woven her story and learning into the words on these pages.

I commend this book to you and pray it will touch your heart as it has touched mine. Whatever lies ahead for you and your family, may you remember the promise of Isaiah 43:2—that as you pass through the waters, our faithful God will be with you. He will never let the waters overwhelm you.

Lucinda van der Hart
Journalist and editor

Introduction

The road to parenthood may be far from straight. For many couples, it is fraught with difficulty, uncertainty and a good deal of heartbreak. The journey to that positive pregnancy test result alone can be a long and complicated one, with plenty of bumps in the road, yet this is just the beginning of the story. For some, there might be a very different path to travel, one that leads to fostering or adoptive parenthood.

Our own journey into parenthood was not straightforward. We went through plenty of heartache, prayers and anguish before we had even conceived. Unaware that I had polycystic ovaries, we endured several years of unexplained infertility until the condition was diagnosed. Then began the path of medical consultations and treatment. There were so many times when we needed great patience and strength from God, while also crying out to him and asking, 'Why isn't it happening, Lord? When will it be our turn?' It was a time of testing, both medically and spiritually, as individuals and as a couple, and of seeking the love, support and prayer of our family and friends when we finally shared our struggle.

Amid our longing for a child and the monthly disappointment and questioning, we somehow managed to become stronger as a couple. We resolved, with a conscious effort, that the huge potential for ongoing stress would not overtake our lives or break us apart. We remained adamant about this, even at our lowest points, even though the strong desire to become parents remained very much in the forefront of our minds. We had countless moments, as we went through this time of waiting and hoping, when we felt powerless and all we could do was rely on God's strength and grace. We knew that we couldn't let our sense of lack steal our joy or prevent us enjoying all the other blessings in our life and our relationship as a couple.

We tried (with varying degrees of success) to maintain this balance when our journey into pregnancy and parenthood finally began. We even had some amusing moments along the way, as we were so resolutely determined not to let the very real stress of the circumstances overwhelm us. One of the most amusing, yet terribly serious, moments that we still smile about was the delivery of a certain sample to be tested (which came back with no irregularities, before the root of our problem was discovered to be my polycystic ovaries). With all the poignant drama and hilarity of a scene from a romantic comedy film, we made the dramatic dash to drop it off on Comic Relief day, of all days. Upon arrival at the fertility department, I was greeted by a lady who was utterly professional and appropriate in her manner. However, she looked uncannily like Dawn French and, in addition to her white lab coat, was wearing red-nose glittery deely-boppers.

Having discovered the cause of our infertility, our prayers were answered after nearly four years, when I became pregnant within a month of having an operation on my ovaries. Our journey to pregnancy had been a rollercoaster and our path into parenthood was only just beginning.

Pregnancy is often not the idyllic or serene time we envisage. Even through illness, anxious times and all the uncertainty we experience as we await our new arrival, we can find God and draw near to him in a new way. The thoughts and reflections that you read in the pages of *Prayer Journey into Parenthood* began life as a series of letters, written throughout my first pregnancy, to our unborn baby 'Pip' (so called because when we found out I was pregnant, after four years of infertility, he was the size of an apple pip). These letters were followed by the reflections I had as a new parent, when I found I was discovering new ways to meet with God in my changing circumstances.

When my first baby was born, I felt an increasingly strong sense of the parallels between my experiences of parenthood and my faith journey. I connected with God in a very different way in those early days of parenthood, and he spoke to me through the daily experiences, despite my extreme tiredness—or perhaps because of it. With hormones and emotions upside down, I somehow managed to find God in powerful words, thoughts and small yet significant moments. In the midst of new circumstances, I had moments when I felt incredibly creative and inspired by God. However, far from being a 'superwoman', I also went through huge trials as I recovered physically, adjusting to parenthood and the emotional turmoil of new choices and responsibilities. It was far from plain sailing.

When I was writing the first draft of this book, in the early days of parenthood the second time around, I felt as inspired and as exhausted as I think it was possible for me to feel, experiencing many moments of utter joy and great trepidation at the same time. God definitely gave me the words I needed as I developed these ideas, when I couldn't have done it in my own strength. Looking back over the writing I did then (often at some very random hours of the day and night, between baby feeds), I genuinely do not recollect composing some of it myself. I can only think that God guided and inspired me at this time, and I give him full credit for his grace at work through me in these pages.

There are many wonderful books already written on parenting or raising your child in faith. The idea behind the development of this book was to offer a different focus, as a devotional aid for parents-to-be as they journey into parenthood. Each of my reflections on the prayer journey parallels the changes, joys and concerns of this season in our walk with God. The book moves stage-by-stage from the positive pregnancy test through to the early days of parenthood, including Bible verses and prayers to support you as you struggle to find quiet moments with God. It is deliberately undated, not to be approached as daily readings but to be picked up whenever you have the time.

How to use *Prayer Journey into Parenthood*

Prayer Journey into Parenthood is designed to be a gentle, supportive companion through your pregnancy and into the early days of new parenthood. It includes chronological devotionals for each stage of the journey, to be read and used to help you along, as and when you feel able, with no pressure. It can be used by expectant mums or those taking steps towards fostering or adoption, and it can be explored together by a couple, to support them both on their shared path into parenthood in relationship with God. The book is written primarily to be read by new mums but is certainly not intended to exclude husbands or partners. It would be an ideal way for expectant parents to reflect together on the way to parenthood and to share precious time as a couple, drawing close to God and seeking him.

If you are using the book with a partner, where the wording says 'I', simply read it as 'we', and consider the devotionals in the context of a partnership. When and how you use the book is up to you, whether you set a particular time aside together or alone, whether you read the chapters in order or dip in and out when you want to reflect on a particular theme.

Devotionals

These begin from the positive pregnancy test and cover a range of experiences, throughout the journey of pregnancy or preparation to foster or adopt, into early parenthood. They also give the opportunity to focus your thoughts back on your continuing faith journey with God, with a parallel Christian theme that allows you to draw near to him.

Bible verses

Each entry suggests some relevant Bible verses to look up and consider. You can read around these verses or look up your own favourite scriptures that spring to mind. You may want to look into further Bible study on some of the themes, if you feel so led. The verses are intended as an encouragement to read God's word and find strength or develop in knowledge, even in the middle of this busy season of change.

Prayer

There is a short written prayer at the end of each devotional. The prayers are intended only as a suggestion, but you may find them helpful. You can read them in silence or aloud. I would encourage you to use them as a springboard for your own prayers for your baby, bringing to God your own journey of faith as you contemplate the themes raised.

Journal space

You may be used to keeping a journal to write down your thoughts and prayers, or it may be something you've never tried. At the end of each devotional, there are several lines left blank, and the way you use them (or not) is entirely up to you. You might find you want to record some details about your current stage of pregnancy or parenthood, as a diary entry, or perhaps you will write a message or letter to your baby. The space can be used for writing down a prayer, your hopes, worries or joys, or Bible verses.

You can even do some doodling if you feel inspired. If you are a prolific writer, you could keep a separate notepad, in order to journal further.

Whether you use *Prayer Journey into Parenthood* by yourself or share the experience with your partner or a family member, it can then be kept as a keepsake. It will be a record of your prayers and thoughts, hopes and concerns as you journeyed through pregnancy, preparing to meet your child, into early parenthood. Looking over your journal notes later can be a wonderful way to remind yourself of prayers that were answered and worries overcome, and of the ways in which you developed in this season, both as a parent-to-be and in your walk with God.

Plenty of trial and error is involved in growing into the role of a parent. Much of the wisdom in this book was picked up as we went along, often worried that we were not doing the right things at all. At times, we genuinely had no idea what to do, and we still feel like that quite regularly, even having done it all again with our second baby. In writing these devotionals I am certainly not suggesting that I am an expert on parenting or that pregnancy or having a newborn baby is easy. The inspiration for this book and the heartfelt reflections I share are firmly rooted in quite the opposite feeling, and a passionate belief in the great need to encourage one another in the journey.

It is my prayer and hope, as you use this book, that it meets you in your need and elation, reassures you and helps you remain close to God as you travel your own amazing, bewildering and joyful road into parenthood.

Section One

PRAYER JOURNEY
THROUGH PREGNANCY

------ *A positive* ------

Your journey into parenthood begins with that nervous, exciting moment as you wait to see a positive pregnancy test. For us, it came after many years of monthly discouragements and a few negative tests taken in hope, before we finally got that long-awaited +.

Take some time to savour the joy of discovering you are pregnant. The huge range of emotions at this precious moment is something to remember and treasure, even if you are also feeling overwhelmed as the reality of the news sinks in.

You may have finally begun the process of moving towards adoption or fostering. Take a moment to appreciate the significance and sense of anticipation that this news brings. It may well have come after many struggles and disappointments, false alarms, medical treatment and possibly even loss. Allow yourself some precious time to stop and revel in this positive news.

Do you remember the joy of first knowing God in a real way, or the moment you gave your life to him and began afresh? You probably felt a similar sense of the enormity of the life-changing experience. Reflect on that positive moment and the powerful emotions of elation and joy that it held. Then consider other pivotal moments in your life and journey with God. Recollect that joy again now, as you praise him for this news and the gift of new life.

BIBLE VERSES
Psalm 139:13 and 2 Corinthians 5:17

Dear Lord, thank you for the joy of this good news! Be with me in all the array of feelings in these first moments of rejoicing and nervous excitement. Praise you for the gift of life—the life you bless me with as I follow you, and this new life forming within me or the child you are preparing me to welcome as an adoptive or foster parent.

Thank you for the day when I began my journey with you. Help me to reflect on the good news of your love for me and to experience a renewed sense of joy in knowing you as my Saviour, as I share this precious moment of discovery with you. May I know a real sense of your presence with me as I take in this news and begin a new chapter of my life. May I know that you are there to guide and comfort me as I start my journey into parenthood. Amen

------ *Patience* ------

Now that you have discovered you are pregnant, there begins a time of waiting. A joyful, yet sometimes anxious first trimester has already begun, a time of great anticipation and wonder. The reality of your pregnancy may not fully have sunk in; alternatively, you may be getting symptoms that make it very apparent, even in these early days.

As you wait for the first scan, it can seem a lifetime away, and it can be hard to imagine the developments going on inside you, if still feel unchanged. You might have begun to read about the miraculous growth your tiny foetus is experiencing, even though you have yet to show any dramatic outward signs of its presence. This can be a quite surreal stage. It is also a time when you need to find peace and patience as you ponder the unseen miracle forming inside you.

I had a strong sense of wanting to enjoy the pregnancy journey and the moments along the way, yet twelve weeks seemed such a long time to wait for that first glimpse. In this initial stage, you can feel as if there is a long road of uncertainty between that positive test and your baby's arrival.

Reflecting on the growth of your unseen baby before the first scan, this is a good time to think about the incredible, unseen growth that has happened within you as you have journeyed with God. From the germination of the tiniest mustard seed of faith, contemplate the ways you have grown and the changes God has made in your heart. Take some moments to ask him to help you to trust him afresh. Seek him for patience as you wait for your baby and for patience in those other life-situations where prayers have not yet been answered. Trust in God's care, in the unseen miracle of your pregnancy, in the road ahead to parenthood and in the path of your whole life. God has it all mapped out, but sometimes we need to rest in this knowledge, enjoy the blessings and experiences of today, and pray for patience as we wait.

Father God, you know the end from the beginning; you are the incredible Creator God. It is not always easy for us to wait patiently or to have faith in something we cannot yet see. Lord, as I wait for a first sight of the invisible miracle that is taking shape within me, help me to trust you. Thank you that you have shaped and changed me from within, and I pray that you would help me to be patient and to trust you with all aspects of my life. Forgive me for the times when I am impatient to see answers. Help me to rest in the reassurance of your love and the paths you have set out for me. I pray that as I wait, you would help me to see the blessings in the present moment. Amen

A wonderful secret

Since finding out that you are pregnant, as the weeks progress you are probably starting to get some symptoms and to feel 'different'. As I've mentioned, I named my tiny miracle 'Pip', having read that, at five weeks' gestation, our baby was the size of an apple pip. This name stuck throughout the pregnancy, as we'd decided to wait until the birth to find out the gender, and it felt so much more personal to use a name rather than referring to our unborn child as 'it'.

You may have been bursting to tell your friends, your family and the rest of the world ever since you've known. However, like us, you may have chosen to wait until you've had your first scan and are through the first trimester before sharing your exciting news. This can be a time of much anticipation, anxiety and even guilty feelings, as you keep your wonderful 'secret'. You may have to avoid questions from your nearest and dearest, those you would usually share everything with. Some eagle-eyed friends and family members may guess or at least suspect your condition and will need to be sworn to secrecy, as you begin avoiding certain foods or opting for soft drinks and decaffeinated alternatives. You may be unusually tired, uncharacteristically emotional or looking rather green around the gills. Quite frankly, you may be simply terrible at keeping a secret and give the news away by a look or smile, or because you just want to shout it from the rooftops. It can be such a special time as you reflect on this greatest piece of news.

When Mary heard the news that she was going to be the mother of Jesus, she took time to reflect on this enormous secret and all that it implied. Do you remember how you felt when you heard the good news of Jesus or experienced God in your life in a real way for the first time? During this period of great anticipation and joy, take some time to reflect on the excitement of knowing God. How do you share the amazing news of God's love with others? Are there times when you keep your faith secret or are you bursting to tell the world the amazing news of salvation?

BIBLE VERSES
Luke 2:19 and 4:43

Dear Lord, while I wait to share the exciting news of impending parenthood, or as I begin to tell those closest to me, help me to use this time to reflect. Help me to give thanks for the incredible blessing of new life, and to think upon the work you are doing within me that is, as yet, a secret. Help me, though, not to keep quiet about your love and grace in my life. I praise you, Lord, for the wonderful news of salvation and the joy of being able to tell the world this news. Help me to find ways to tell others about your presence in my life and not to keep you secret. May I find opportunities and have the confidence to speak of your goodness and faithfulness. Amen

------ *First sight* ------

Seeing your baby for the first time at your first scan is awesome; it is quite incredible to see that tiny person beginning to take shape. However many times you have seen it on television or in films, to look at a scan of the tiny human being who is forming inside you seems miraculous. Although it is not the clearest of images and the baby is a long way from looking like a fully formed person, this remains one of the most significant and emotional moments to treasure during early pregnancy. It is amazing to think how much the baby has grown already in twelve weeks, and to imagine the changes still to come.

You may have felt a whole range of emotions as you finally saw the scan image—relief, joy, excitement and perhaps some degree of anxiety or fear at the enormity of this event and the implications of the journey ahead. You are likely to be feeling overwhelmed, praising God for the miracle you have now seen with your own eyes, the miracle of creation now really visible in its early stages of growth. The relief and joy at seeing our baby for the first time, being reassured that all was OK and seeing that tiny heart beat, was breathtaking. It was after our first scan that I began to write a series of letters to Pip, our long-awaited first child, recounting how he was already showing signs of being a little individual—such as refusing to lie the 'right' way up for the sonographer.

Think about a time when you have seen God at work in your life or the lives of others, perhaps for the first time. When have you seen with your own eyes a clear manifestation of his power, presence and grace in your life? When have you had a significant realisation of the awesomeness of his creation? Reflect on the early days of walking with him, perhaps remembering afresh the life-changing moment when you saw clearly for the first time and began your journey with God.

BIBLE VERSE
Jeremiah 1:5

Creator God, thank you for the wonder of seeing my baby for the first time. I praise you for the journey so far and the work you are doing within me as the miracle of growth continues. Thank you that, at twelve weeks, this tiny miracle is now visible. I give you thanks for the joy of this moment of first sight and ask that you would be with me in all the emotions that go with this amazing reality. Help me to remember afresh the sense of awe and wonder I felt when I first beheld your love and power in my life.

Forgive me for the times when I forget the unseen and visible wonders of your creation and the way you are evident in my life. Help me to remember those incredible moments when you have been tangible and real in my life and the lives of others. Lord, I seek to see you more and experience a new vision of your greatness at this significant time. Amen

Proud parents already

Now that you have seen your little miracle, you are probably sharing your scan picture on social media, showing it to everyone and repeatedly looking at that treasured image. Despite the fact that the picture may look rather more like a kidney bean than a baby, to you it is the most incredible thing you've ever seen and you can't help but share your delight. When my sister-in-law showed my niece our scan picture, she promptly declared that it looked more like a small kitten than a baby and asked if we were sure it wasn't one. Given that Pip had spent most of the time curled up asleep during the scan, we could see what she meant.

Although others will be incredibly pleased and excited for you, this image will probably not evoke the same level of elation and wonder in everyone as it does in you. You gaze at the tiny beginnings of an actual person who is taking shape within you. In this grainy photo you see a wonderful miracle—your baby, a new person like no other before.

When God looks at you, he sees the most incredible creation, too. Just like a proud parent-to-be marvelling at that first image, he loves you, whatever shape you are in. Regardless of how you feel about yourself, your appearance, your flaws and failings, God sees a work of art, a beautiful wonder of his creation. Perhaps you are far from feeling like a fully grown, well-developed Christian, but God looks at you and sees a miracle. You are his child. You may have much growing and developing yet to do, but to him you are marvellous.

Take some time to consider this, and believe that God, your heavenly Father, loves you and delights in what he sees—not because you are perfect, but because he knows you. He created you and he sees the potential you have within you. God does not make mistakes; nor does he reject his children, however much they have sinned and however many times you feel you have fallen short or are unworthy of his love. He sees his marvellous creation and he is pleased—a very proud parent.

BIBLE VERSES
Isaiah 43:4 and Ephesians 2:10

Father God, thank you for the small person who is changing and developing daily in my womb. I praise you for the chance to see an image of my child and I ask that you will be with me as I begin to feel parental pride and joy.

Thank you that you see me, your child, as a wonder of your creation—a masterpiece. You do not see me as I see myself. Thank you that you love me despite my flaws and can see the potential for me to be the person that you created me to be. I pray that you would help me believe that I am loved, made in your image and beautiful in your sight. Help me to trust in the changing power of your loving grace. Forgive me when I fall short of all that I can be, and help me to see myself as you see me, as a new creation. Amen

------ *Telling the world* ------

The time has come when you are telling everyone you know (and possibly anyone else who will listen) about your pregnancy. You have been longing to share this wonderful news and are thrilled to announce your pregnancy to the world. You may well have come up with a clever or poignant way of revealing your impending parenthood. Perhaps, though, you have just quietly told those you love, who are rejoicing with you after a long road leading to this most wonderful announcement.

I remember well how delighted our family and friends were when we finally told them we were expecting our first child, after many years of hoping and praying. We announced the news of our second baby with the scan picture on social media, but first we had fun at our elder son's second birthday party by dressing him in a T-shirt that read 'I'm going to be a big brother!' for a surprise double celebration as people eventually spotted it. Take some time to appreciate this important time of celebration, to savour the special gift of being able to share such happy news, now that the secret is out.

Do you remember sharing the good news of Jesus with others for the first time? Did you quietly tell the people who are close to you? Perhaps you were bursting with uncontainable joy and felt like shouting the news from the rooftops. Just like the wonderful news of becoming pregnant, our joy at knowing Jesus in our life can be expressed in many ways. It can also bring a mixture of emotions as it provides a completely new view of the world. Your journey of faith may have started at the end of a road fraught with twists and turns, a path paved with years of searching, heartache, hope or pain. You may need to take some time to acknowledge that journey into relationship with God, but then leave it firmly in your past as you remember again the good news and joy of freedom through Christ.

Perhaps you feel that, in all honesty, your excitement and awe have dimmed over time; you no longer feel the burning desire to tell the world about God's saving grace. Bring to God your honest feelings, without fear of recrimination, and reflect once more on the good news of Jesus.

BIBLE VERSES
Psalm 51:12 and Matthew 28:19–20

Saviour God, thank you for the blessing of being able to share the incredible news of this pregnancy with unbridled joy and rejoicing. Help me to remember and appreciate anew the freedom and wonder I found when I began my walk with you. Restore in me the feelings of hope and courage that need rekindling, and give me opportunities to share the good news of your love.

I pray that as I share, happily and confidently, the news of my growing baby, you would help me to use this time to tell others the news not only of this wonderful blessing but also of your great mercy and love, Creator God. Help me to take the chance to tell the great news of knowing you as Saviour. Amen

_____

_____

_____

_____

_____

_____

_____

_____

_____

_____

What's in a name?

Choosing a name for your baby is an exciting task. It can also feel like a very big responsibility when you consider that this will be your child's identity as they grow. You may be reading lots of lists or buying books to search for the perfect name that you will love. This process can be the focus of many discussions and even arguments as you try to reach a decision. Do you choose something with a special meaning or significance? Is there a name that is traditional in your family? What will others think of your choice? We managed to agree upon a girl's name many years before we became pregnant, yet it took us quite some time to settle upon boys' names during both pregnancies. Fortunately we managed it eventually, as we are sure neither of our boys would have appreciated the girl's name we picked.

Your name is such a huge part of who you are. It's the way others identify you, whether you like the name that was chosen for you or not. God knows your name. Not only that, but he knows all about you—your personality, hopes, triumphs and failings. Many names in the Bible have special meanings or are chosen for particular reasons, and many parents-to-be take inspiration from scripture when searching for a suitable and meaningful name for a child. The name Jesus, for example, means 'God saves' and was chosen before his birth by God. This most significant of names was both his identity and the basis of his mission on earth. There are many other names for Jesus, used to describe his personality and what he meant to those who met him. For example, he is known as Emmanuel (God with us), healer, teacher, king, redeemer, saviour and friend.

Reflect on these names for Jesus and what he means to you. What is his identity in your life? What does it mean to you, to find your purpose and identity through a relationship with Christ? You may have perceived Jesus in terms of differing facets of his personality during significant times in your life. It is quite likely that you would call him by a name quite different from the one someone else would use to describe who he is to them.

God knows your name and everything about you. Your name is written on his hand; you are significant and valued. Your name is 'child of God'; your identity is secure in him. God knows and loves you.

BIBLE VERSE
Isaiah 49:16

Father God, thank you that you know me by name. Help me to remember that you love me and know all about me—not only my name, but my hopes and fears, my joys and sorrows. Help me to reflect afresh today on the amazing name of you—Jesus, my God, my Lord and Saviour.

Father, King, Healer, Redeemer, Teacher and Friend—as I say and meditate upon these descriptions of you, may I appreciate their meaning to me and bring you praise as I worship you through prayer. Amen

------ *Hearing that heart beat* ------

Hearing your baby's heart beat for the first time is not only reassuring beyond words but can be one of the most incredible moments of amazement. Seeing your baby on a scan image makes your pregnancy feel more 'real' and is astounding. However, certainly at the first scan, your baby still looks only just recognisable as a small person. When you actually hear that rapid, determined little heartbeat, it is a hugely emotional experience of life within your womb. A heartbeat is a universally distinguishable, vital sign of life. When I was able to hear this mindblowing rhythm for the very first time, at our 16-week midwife's visit, it was amazing. I was relieved when the midwife found it with ease, and it was a joy to hear after all the medical drama involved in getting to this stage with Pip.

Do you recall the first time you felt a real sense of knowing God's heart of love for you? Perhaps there have been other significant moments in your faith journey, when you have sensed his presence in a way that was powerful yet comforting, like the sound of a heartbeat. Seeking God's will involves taking time to stop, reflect and engage in listening for his 'heart'. This might be done by reading his word, inviting him to speak to you through scripture, by immersing yourself in the words of worship songs, or perhaps through the teaching and actions of others. Sometimes we need to spend time simply resting in his presence, drawing near to him and being open to hear from him. His love for us beats as strongly as a heartbeat, providing the lifeblood and energy we need in our daily life to empower us with his strength and Holy Spirit.

Consider the ways in which you have known this closeness with God. How do you find his 'heart' and draw near to him? Take some time to rest, asking God for a fresh experience of him as you seek him. Lay your life and heart open to him. Find a way that is comfortable to you, and confidently draw near in anticipation to know his heart and hear from him.

BIBLE VERSES
1 Chronicles 16:11 and 1 Kings 19:12

Dear Lord, thank you that it is possible to hear the heartbeat of a tiny, growing baby. I praise you for this marvel of creation and for the reassurance of hearing that irrefutable evidence of vital life and energy within. Help me to seek to know and hear your heart for me—the still small voice that whispers words of hope and comfort, or the pounding thunder of the strength of your love for me, by which your Son overcame death to set me free. Help me to draw near to you with a thankful heart as I reflect on the amazing sound of my baby's heartbeat. May I find ways to spend time giving you the chance to impart to me your 'heart', to know your love and grace through your Holy Spirit and to rest in your presence. Amen

First flutters

Feeling your baby move for the first time is amazing, especially if this is your first pregnancy. Physically experiencing those little wriggly feelings and realising that they are coming not from your stomach but from the baby is so very exciting and strange. It is a reassuring and much-anticipated sensation, but it may happen a few times before you are sure that it's your baby starting to get active. It will be a long while until the kicks are strong enough to be felt and seen by anyone but you, but these first flutters are a truly astounding stage of bonding as your baby grows and makes its presence felt. Feeling these movements helps you connect with the little being who is developing in your care. I remember describing it as like the sensation of a mobile phone vibrating inside me—a curious feeling.

Your experience of becoming a Christian may have begun with a very dramatic encounter with God, or it may have been a slow realisation of what God meant to you and the ways in which he was apparent in your daily life. As we continue our journey of growth in faith, it is often a slow process. Some things change dramatically and instantly when we invite God to inhabit our life and renew our mind, but others change gradually, deep within us. You may have found yourself responding to God and experiencing a change in your mindset or making a conscious effort to think about your words and actions. These changes may not have been instantly noticeable to the people around you, but you felt a change as you invited God into your heart and asked him to move in your life.

Take some time to reflect on those early stages of change in you as a Christian. Just like those first baby movements, it is these changes that make the living out of our faith start to feel more 'real' as we invite God to help us grow and actively change from within. How does your faith feel evident in your life now? Do you still feel within you those movements of God? Do you need to ask God for a fresh experience of those first 'flutters' of realisation that he can change our hearts and mind?

```
BIBLE VERSE
1 Corinthians 3:16
```

Dear Lord, thank you for the incredible joy of feeling my baby begin to move. Those first wriggling sensations are amazing. Thank you that you dwell within my being and can move within me too, gently yet perceivably. Help me to take some time to appreciate afresh those gentle, bubbling signs of your presence. Forgive me for times when I do not seek you or invite you to continue to help me develop a renewed heart. Help me to feel a fresh sense of your being at work within me at this time, and help me to know how to make changes in my thoughts and actions that might make your presence more evident in my daily life. Amen

Antenatal antics

Antenatal classes can be daunting, fun and quite bizarre. Meeting other parents-to-be who are going through similar experiences (and yet who may be very different in their thinking), to learn about birth and parenting, can be illuminating. It can also be amusing, reassuring and heartening to share this part of the pregnancy journey with others and to have the opportunity to ask questions and seek guidance from the class leader. Some of the facts about birth, along with all the information and practical tips about caring for a newborn, can be overwhelming and scary. We found the classes to be informative as well as a great environment in which to be vulnerable and honest about fears and lack of knowledge. This shared experience at such a significant time in your life can often lead to friendships that develop after your babies are born. At the very least, you may meet some of your fellow novice parents at the hospital once your babies have been delivered, so you can discover how things went for them and introduce your new arrivals.

In our faith-life, as we begin to learn and grow as Christians, the support and shared experience of meeting with our church family or Christian friends can help us enormously as we seek to develop in our knowledge of the faith. Much like those antenatal classes, finding a church or group of Christian friends with whom we can be vulnerable and engage in teaching and worship is a huge part of nurturing our growth. Like having care from a variety of medical professionals, seeking support and advice from Christian leaders or trusted friends is significant in supporting and nurturing our spiritual well-being. Meeting with a small group or the wider church family, and praying and learning together in a safe and caring environment, helps us in all areas of life, both personally and spiritually. Finding people you trust and can seek out for advice and prayer support is particularly crucial as you journey through your pregnancy and early parenthood. They can help you adapt to these life-changes as you continue to develop in faith and understanding on your journey with God.

BIBLE VERSE
1 Thessalonians 5:11

Dear Lord, thank you for the people you have placed into our lives to support and encourage us and to walk with us at this time of change and learning, on the journey to parenthood. Thank you for the chance to meet with other parents-to-be, to share in the nervous anticipation of this big life-change and to have fun learning together and asking questions. Thank you that, as Christians, we can also seek advice, support and friendship from our church family or from Christian friends and leaders.

I pray that, in this time of learning and growth, you would help me remember to ask for the prayers and guidance of people I trust, both for the pregnancy and parenting journey still ahead and for my spiritual growth and well-being. Help me to ask questions, to seek you and not to be afraid to ask for prayer and learn from other Christians. Amen

Amazing growth

It is marvellous, week by week, to realise all the complex changes that your baby is going through. This miraculous growth happens in tiny but remarkable ways, from the moment a child is conceived. It is a wonder of God's creation and mindblowing in its intricacy. Some books and websites that document the stages of a baby's development compare its increasing size to different pieces of fruit. From the size of an apple pip at five weeks, the baby reaches approximately the size of a grape at nine weeks and, by the 20-week mark, is about as big as a banana. I was fascinated by these comparisons to fruit and I recorded the rough comparative sizes in my letters to Pip. I was amazed afresh, during my second pregnancy, by how quickly we reached the 'grape' stage.

Our faith can often feel small to us—even embryonic, very far from the size we would like it to be. However, even if our faith is as tiny as a mustard seed, God's word tells us, we can do amazing things when we entrust our growth to him. Just like a developing baby, our faith grows with each tiny step we take with God.

Consider the steps of growth you have made over time in your walk with God. Some may seem minuscule and insignificant, and others huge and life-changing. Do not dismiss even the most inconsequential-seeming step of change; each and every moment has contributed to your growth and every experience has helped to shape you into the person you are now.

BIBLE VERSE
Matthew 17:20

Creator God, thank you for the incredible stages of growth that are happening week by week. Thank you that I can imagine my baby's size and even see pictures of the tiny but wonderful changes that are going on.

Thank you that you have been with me at each small stage of growth that I have made in my walk with you. Forgive me when I forget that these small steps of faith really are significant. Help me to keep taking opportunities to grow and mature in my faith-life. Whatever stage of development I am at in my journey with you, God, help me to trust in you and to continue to change and learn, not to stay the same size.

When my faith feels tiny and the mountains in my way seem immovable, help me to bring them to you. I entrust my life and faith, however fragile or insignificant they may feel, into your hands afresh. Help me to believe and trust that you, the God who created me and the miracle that is growing within me, can do immeasurably more than I can even imagine. Amen

Baby talk

It can seem strange to talk to your baby bump; perhaps you feel a little self-conscious or silly. Maybe, though, you have naturally chattered to your growing baby from the moment you knew they were there. I found I automatically began speaking to my baby; although it felt odd at first, it soon became very natural to talk to this little person. I began quietly, with just thoughts in my head; then I started to voice an occasional conspiratorial whispered greeting of 'Hello in there!' while my pregnancy was not yet public knowledge. I then progressed to telling Pip all kinds of things, and eventually to feeling my baby move in response to my voice.

Some parents-to-be are entirely comfortable narrating their daily activities, telling their unborn baby all about the world, who they will meet when they arrive in the family, and so on. It can be a fantastic way of bonding with your baby during pregnancy. Conversely, as you busily continue with normal life, perhaps you are only now adjusting to the idea of pregnancy or have been feeling so unwell that it hasn't even occurred to you to talk to your developing baby. There are no rights or wrongs and the baby will become familiar with your voice as you speak to others. It is certainly a precious feeling to know that your baby can hear you.

When we bring our daily life before God in prayer, he wants our words to reflect our love for him and to be honest and heartfelt. God does not need our prayers to be complicated; they can be as easy as a conversation with someone standing right there with you, someone to whom you can happily relate your worries, hopes and joys. It is great to spend time talking to God, perhaps bringing to him very detailed prayers of thanksgiving and intercession, and admitting to him our failings or needs. However, God wants us simply to share our hearts, just as we communicate with our unborn baby. He wants us to pray with integrity in a way that feels comfortable, giving him praise and inviting him to be at the centre of our daily life.

BIBLE VERSES
1 John 5:14–15 and Matthew 6:6–8

Dear God, thank you that when we pray, whether it's with others or in the privacy and rawness of our hearts, you hear us. Forgive me when I forget to invite you into my daily life, when I feel constrained by the desire to have the 'right' words, when I am weary in body or soul or when the words just will not come. Help me to know afresh that the words I say are not as important as the laying before you of my life, my cares and my joys, simply asking you to draw close to me. May my prayers be acceptable and pleasing to your ears, Lord. Just like the baby beginning to hear and recognise my voice, may I realise that I am known and familiar to you and that you delight in every prayer from me, your child. Amen

------ *Food for thought* ------

There is so much said about what you can and can't eat or drink during pregnancy. There are also plenty of foods you might either crave or begin to dislike as your body adjusts to pregnancy. You might feel overwhelmed by the advice you are bombarded with or by the responsibility of 'feeding' your baby a healthy diet. Perhaps you simply feel too sick to keep much food down at all. Although I didn't suffer too badly with morning sickness, I remember that citrus drinks helped, and I took a particular liking to barbecue flavour crisps, as I could face them when I felt too ill to eat anything else. On the other hand, I went completely off the taste of milky tea.

Adjusting to the guidelines about what is 'safe' to eat when pregnant can be quite daunting. Particularly with your first pregnancy, you will probably keep checking, for example, whether a certain cheese is OK if cooked or not, and you'll take steps to avoid alcohol and caffeine in quantity. This alone may be a tough adjustment to make.

We can feel that our spiritual 'food' habits are similarly complex or hard to get to grips with. We are faced with so many different interpretations of scripture that we are left unsure how to get a balanced spiritual diet to help us to grow and develop in faith. Taking advice from trusted Christian friends or leaders and seeking God's wisdom can help us to discern what is good for us to 'digest' in our walk with God, and what to avoid or give up.

Take some time to think about the spiritual food you take in on a daily basis. Are you absorbing teaching that helps you to grow, that edifies and encourages you in your faith, yet is also challenging and gives you food for thought? Do you find that you are easily distracted by opinions or teachings that leave you confused? Perhaps you have neglected to seek a diet of prayer, worship and teaching that nourishes you spiritually, and you need to look at ways to get the balance right again. Consider the steps you could take to get back to those healthy basics. Take time to find spiritual nourishment from God's word, the teaching of others and the support and prayer of trusted Christian friends or leaders.

BIBLE VERSES
Psalm 34:8 and John 4:31–34

Father God, thank you that we can find nourishment for our soul in your word. Thank you that you provide for our growth and spiritual health, just as I strive to feed my growing baby what is healthy and good during pregnancy. Help me not to worry excessively about the diet changes required during this time, but to seek advice and to take sensible steps where required. Forgive me when I overcomplicate my spiritual diet, and help me to know what is nourishing for my spiritual well-being and what is not. Help me to find ways to get some basic spiritual food into my daily life, if I have slipped into a less enriching diet, and help me to rediscover a healthy balance of prayer, teaching and support from other Christians. Amen

------ *Singing to baby* ------

Babies can hear from about 29 weeks and are then able to respond to sounds, so your voice, music and other loud sounds can cause them to wriggle. It is fantastic to feel them kick or move in response to music or when you or someone else talks to them. Playing music or singing to your baby is fun and it helps you feel a connection to the little character who is developing, ready to become part of your family. Babies will begin to recognise your voice and the voices of people they hear often. You may feel self-conscious singing to your baby or playing your favourite tunes. However, it is not silly and babies don't care how good a singer you are: they just love to hear your familiar voice and they react to the movement it causes within your body.

I remember my babies wriggling when I sang in church or played my favourite songs around the house. It was also a source of much merriment when my husband made up funny personalised songs to sing to my bump during pregnancy. It was a special part of bonding as, over time, the baby started responding with movement to his voice too.

Just like a growing baby, God delights in hearing us sing or play songs of worship and adoration to him. Like your baby, God does not judge your ability to hold a note; he doesn't listen to your singing with a critical ear. He is not sitting in judgement on your 'talent' or analysing it for its pitch. Nor does your heavenly Father compare your worship to that of others; he simply delights to hear you bring your honest, heartfelt praise to him.

Making a joyful sound is about more than just the noise we create; it is a reflection of our heart. The Lord does not want us to sing or make music to impress others. It is the worship we offer with genuine feeling that is most pleasing to God—an overflowing expression of our love, thankfulness or need for God's strength and grace. It does not matter to God if we sing with a clear and confident voice, as long as our worship is poured out of a heart of love and adoration.

BIBLE VERSES
Psalm 95:1 and 100:1–2

Dear Lord, thank you that I can sing to my baby even while they are in the womb, and that they can appreciate and respond to my voice. How amazing it is that my growing baby can take delight in music already. I pray that my worship would be pleasing to your ear. May you hear my heartfelt praise and worship, not just words or a performance. Help me to bring my worship to you with confidence, knowing that you accept it. Thank you, Lord, that you do not judge us as the world does but are pleased when we bring our offerings of worship to you. Amen

Anxious times

Pregnancy is a time not only filled with joyful anticipation but also fraught with anxieties, uncertainty and, at times, abject fear and panic. However much they try to be calm and take everything in their stride, even the most cool and collected parent-to-be will experience a massive range of new worries and thoughts. A whole host of anxieties and questions (both logical and illogical) about your baby and yourself combine to perplex and concern you as you journey through the uncharted sea that is pregnancy. It is often overwhelming, dealing with thoughts about the future as you try to prepare for all that is ahead while handling the many emotional fluctuations and uncertainties of this current season of life.

Having waited for so long to become pregnant, I was overjoyed finally to be carrying my child, but I still had to trust this precious little being, consciously and frequently, to God's care, as each concern arose about his well-being, movements and so on. It would have been easy to let the very natural worries of a first-time parent-to-be diminish the joy. It is far too easy, in many areas of life, to let the unknown or the possibility of 'what might happen' in a given circumstance overtake us and cast a shadow of worry over our contentment. Doubts, concerns and worries, though very natural responses to important events or seasons in our life, can cloud our perspective and rob us of joy.

What is stopping you from embracing all the excitement and joy of your journey through pregnancy? Take some time to consider the things that make you anxious and bring them to God. Are you worrying, in anticipation, about numerous scenarios that you can do little about until they arrive? This is natural but also futile: you are concerning yourself with potential problems that you may not ever encounter. Make a conscious effort to call to mind Jesus' words in Matthew 6:34 when your worries about the future threaten to overshadow your present blessings.

BIBLE VERSE
Matthew 6:34

Dear Lord, thank you that you are a mighty and powerful God and yet you are interested in every concern and anxiety we have, however insignificant it may seem. Help me to trust you with the things that burden me along each step of the journey of pregnancy and in my daily life. Forgive me when I struggle with worry and forget to seek your peace and guidance. Help me to trust all my tomorrows to you and to give my concerns over to you in prayer. May I find joy in the blessings of this season, knowing you have the present and future in your care. Amen

------ *Visibly blooming* ------

As the weeks go by, your body shape gradually changes until your growing bump is unmistakable. Your pregnancy at this stage becomes visible to the world and it is obvious that you have a baby on board. This can be a wonderful time of 'blooming', with some of the unpleasant symptoms having subsided. You might be enjoying showing off your bump and beginning to feel more energised. Alternatively, perhaps you still feel unwell or tired as you carry around your increasingly weighty and very visible little miracle.

Take some time to rest and get to know your new body shape. Reflect on the incredible process your body is going through as you carry your growing baby and enjoy the good wishes of others. Some people may be so delighted that they ask to touch the bump and feel a kick. This can seem a bit intrusive and you may not be particularly comfortable with it. However, it is also a wonderful expression of other people's desire to share in the exciting experience. I was very proud of my bump and loved wearing maternity clothes, rejoicing in being pregnant, once it was clear that I was not just putting on a bit of extra weight. My favourite top was a T-shirt showing a cartoon of a baby inside the womb, reading a book. As an unashamed bookworm, I loved wearing this T-shirt as my bump grew bigger, and it certainly raised some smiles.

Does your faith 'show' to the world, like your baby bump? Is God's presence in you just as obvious to the people around you? Can others tell when they meet you that there is something different about you because you know Jesus? Do your outward actions, your appearance and the words you speak display your love for God and the compassion he calls us to show to others? Take some time to reflect on the ways your faith is visible. Bring to God the things in your life that you know don't help your faith to be evident to the world. Is your faith growing, blossoming and undeniably obvious, or are there ways in which you need to show your faith more confidently?

BIBLE VERSES
Philippians 4:5 and Micah 6:8

Father God, thank you for the amazing growth of my baby, now so visible. Help me to take time to reflect on the changes to my body shape and to give thanks for the way that my body is keeping this baby safe and protected. Although the changes in my appearance can feel strange and uncomfortable, help me to see the astonishing work that you are doing, equipping my frame to carry my baby.

There are often times when I forget to shine for you, to show in my words, actions and attitudes the love of Christ. Forgive me when my faith is far from 'blooming' and is not reflected in my daily life for all to see. Help me to acknowledge that it isn't always easy and to find ways in which I could act or speak to display your grace and love to others more overtly. Amen

_____

_____

_____

_____

_____

_____

_____

_____

_____

_____

Power from within

Having felt the baby wriggling around inside you for quite some time, it can be a long wait before those movements are strong enough to be felt or seen from the outside. It is a remarkable moment when the people close to you can finally feel a kick or even see your bump move. The size and strength of your growing baby are now unmistakable, as he or she moves around more and becomes more agile. The power exerted by a baby within is sometimes forceful enough to take your breath away, and it is so exciting to share these movements with others. I remember my husband being impatient to feel our baby kick for the first time, and delighted when he could see my bump wriggling. We found it amusing that as we sat watching television, Pip would have a 'dance'; when I settled down to relax, he started partying. The reassuring wriggle each night as I settled to sleep was especially comforting, though not always comfortable.

The strength of God's love and the power of his Holy Spirit are alive within us, just like this growing, active baby. The power that dwells inside us when we invite God into our heart is unseen, yet it should, arguably, be visible and tangible to others. When we experience the transforming love and power of God, the gentle healer, the changes can be gradual or dramatic. We might feel moved to alter our behaviour, attitudes and words in response to the inward change of heart, and with the guidance of God's grace at work in us. Do you think others can see or experience the outward effect of the power of the Holy Spirit within you? Is it evident in the way you live your life?

BIBLE VERSE
Ephesians 1:13

Dear Lord, thank you that as my baby grows in size and kicks more and more, the movements are so very noticeable that they can even be felt from outside. Thank you that although these kicks can be uncomfortable at times, they are reassuring and a wonderful outward sign of the active, determined baby I am carrying. Help me to take time to appreciate the power of your love and grace, powerfully at work within me. Help me to know afresh the power of your Holy Spirit living within me. Forgive me when my words or actions do not display outwardly the love that dwells within me. May the power and strength of your Holy Spirit and your love and grace be visible to those I encounter and be felt in the way I live my daily life. Amen

------ Bump in the road ------

During the journey into parenthood, many unexpected concerns can arise. There might be worrying medical complications for you or the baby or other life events that occur unexpectedly, like a bereavement or other upheaval in your family. If you are travelling the road to fostering or adoption, there will be plenty of different stages in the process and testing times to overcome.

When we discovered with great joy that we were expecting our second son, it was not long after my dad had passed away. On top of these intense mixed emotions, doctors found fluid on our baby's brain at the 20-week scan, and my grandpa's death came shortly afterwards. In the midst of so much worry, grief and additional scans, we had to trust God and seek his strength. In our times of anxiety about what lay ahead, we tried to take things step by step, relying on our faith that God had given us the baby who was meant for us. It was only by the grace of God and the prayer and love of those around us that we coped with all the uncertainty. Miraculously, as it was regularly monitored, the fluid on our baby's brain reduced and the scan that was done the day after his birth showed no fluid at all.

God wants us to bring our lives to him—our good times, our heartache and our illness—and draw near to him. Trusting God with unexpected and painful events isn't easy but he can carry our burdens and wants us to trust him with the bigger picture. Ask him to guide you when the way is not smooth on your road to parenthood. Ideals you held might have been shattered and you may have some very tough situations to endure. Place each step into his care, and be kind to yourself when you feel upset or angry about the complications, or when the journey to parenthood is complex and you feel nothing like the 'glowing' pregnant woman you imagined being. It is far from easy to be patient in affliction, but try to find moments of joy, knowing that God's love and hope remain steadfast. Write down your anxieties and your joys and commit them prayerfully to God, trusting that he is walking with you through the difficult times.

BIBLE VERSE
1 Peter 5:7

Dear God, when difficulties hit me like relentless waves, and unexpected trials or worries threaten my peace, may I seek you more than ever. Help me to process feelings of disappointment when things do not go to plan in my journey or I have to deal with other life situations that overshadow the joys of this season. May I not be overwhelmed when unforeseen events or medical complications make the path ahead unclear. Be with me as I travel a road that wasn't anticipated and help me to bring each step before you. Lord, I pray that your comforting presence would wash over me. May your love, which casts out fear, still my anxious mind and fill my troubled heart with hope to face the journey ahead. Amen

------ *Are you prepared?* ------

It can be a lot of fun getting kitted out, ready for the baby. Shopping for all those important pieces of furniture, practical equipment and adorable outfits is an exciting part of getting ready for your new arrival. The range of choices can be mind-blowing to a first-time parent. You may wonder where to start. How will you know if you have bought the 'best' equipment? Are you prepared for all eventualities? Do you have all the essential little accoutrements as well as the larger pieces? You may have been painstakingly consulting baby magazines and stocking up on things that others have recommended for some time now.

Whether you are pregnant or preparing to welcome your foster or adoptive child into your family, this is a crucial stage of preparation. When we were preparing for our first baby, we thoroughly enjoyed sourcing nursery items to fit our woodland theme, delighted to be able to buy lots of baby products at last. We asked friends and family for their tips on what we should or shouldn't buy. However, in hindsight, not all the things we thought essential were really necessary. Beautiful as our lovingly prepared nursery looked, in practice our newborn refused to nap in his cot and we barely used the mobile that coordinated so well with the room. We also definitely overstocked on cotton wool and scratch mitts.

When it comes to our faith, are we equipping ourselves with the right things? What do you actually *need* to nurture your relationship with God? Our Christian lives can easily get crowded with practices or paraphernalia that seem essential but are not really needed. Take some time to reflect on ways you can simplify your life with God to establish a closer connection with him at the heart of your life. Perhaps start using some new Bible reading notes; or talk to trusted Christian friends or leaders at your church to support you in the changes you want to make. Take time to engage with worship music and prayer in a way that helps you draw close to God. Being prepared to invite Jesus into our life afresh, along with a new baby, means simply opening our hearts. No fancy preparation is required, apart from the basic necessities of a loving heart and open arms.

BIBLE VERSES
Revelation 3:20 and Philippians 4:8

Dear Lord, thank you for the privilege and excitement of preparing all that is needed to welcome and provide for a child. Help me to seek advice and to make sensible choices about what is needed, yet also to enjoy the fun of choosing things for the new arrival.

Forgive me when I overcomplicate my faith-life or listen to confusing or inaccurate teaching, forgetting simply to trust in you and your word. Help me to find ways to rediscover those simple, essential parts of my Christian life that anchor me firmly to you, rather than allowing myself to be distracted by unnecessary things. May I find afresh the heart of worship, seek those who encourage and strengthen me in my faith journey and discern what is 'essential', giving you the central focus in my life. Amen

Growing pains

Your body is adapting in lots of ways, from the moment you conceive, to accommodate your baby. Miraculous as this natural process is, it is not always comfortable and, as your pregnancy progresses, these 'growing pains' can become acute. Your muscles and ligaments relax and stretch in new ways and vital organs are being shifted around within you to make room for your expanding womb and to ensure the baby's comfort. This can cause all kinds of aches and some quite debilitating conditions. During my second pregnancy, I developed a condition that caused chronic pain in my pelvis, hip and back. The situation became so difficult that I was using crutches by the end of my pregnancy and required treatment from a physiotherapist and osteopath to ease the painful symptoms.

Our Christian growth can be painful as we are transformed and moulded by God, the potter. Simply accepting that we need to develop can challenge and stretch us. However, like the changes required to carry a baby safely, the adaptations that may be required when we bring our life to God are worthwhile when we see the end result. Our behaviour, thoughts and attitudes might need serious modification, and this can be a difficult process as we face our faults and failings and ask God to shape us into the person he made us to be. Being questioned by others about our faith or meeting ridicule or opposition can also be a painful, stretching experience. Tough times, in which our faith is hard to live out, can threaten to break us, but they are part of the refining process of being transformed by God's redeeming love.

BIBLE VERSES
Isaiah 64:8 and 2 Corinthians 4:8–12

Father God, thank you for the miraculous changes that my body has undergone to house and protect my growing baby. Help me to seek your comfort and strength when this stretching and growth causes me pain. May I trust my spiritual development into your hands and commit it afresh to you, allowing you to shape and form me. Forgive me when I do not seek to be challenged or to grow in my faith-life but take the more comfortable choices. Help me not to miss opportunities to be moulded by you. Amen

Surrounded by prayer

Prayer is such a central part of our faith, yet so often we forget to include it routinely in our daily life. Perhaps you feel that requesting prayer in church or from a trusted Christian friend is somehow selfish or only for the times of greatest need. The Bible teaches that we should seek God in all things, praying for each other and for our own needs. Pregnancy can be a worrying time, with so much that is unknown or new. Medical problems can cause huge heartache and anxiety. With your baby's birth approaching, you may be feeling nervous, yet you may forget to ask for prayer.

Is there someone you can invite to pray for you and your unborn baby at this time? When some friends organised a 'baby shower' for me, I was delighted but I didn't want it to be just about silly games and gifts for the baby. We organised some fun activities but I also asked some of the women for a 'prayer shower'. It was a really wonderful time of feeling supported and blessed, as well as a gentle witness to my non-Christian guests of the importance of God to me on my journey through pregnancy. I sent each guest home with a candle to light and asked them to pray on the day of my baby's delivery. Due to a retinal condition, I knew I needed to have a planned Caesarean section, so it was comforting to know that my female friends and relatives would be holding me in prayer on this specific day as I moved into parenthood.

It's good to ask someone you trust to pray with you towards the end of pregnancy or to keep you in their prayers for specific concerns as the birth day approaches. Do we ask others to pray for us regularly in our everyday life too?

BIBLE VERSE
Philippians 2:3–4

Dear Lord, thank you that you provide others to support me on the journey into parenthood. Help me to approach trusted Christian friends with confidence and ask them to pray with me or for me as I move through this season of waiting and prepare for the birth of my baby. Forgive me when I forget to bring my hopes, concerns and joys to you daily in prayer. Help me to offer my life and the life of my baby into your care and to continue to ask for your strength and guidance as I become a parent.

------ *Persevering through pain* ------

Pregnancy brings with it a multitude of aches and pains as the baby grows and moves around, especially towards the end. The discomfort of carrying your baby will soon be over, and your thoughts now naturally turn to the goal before you, the impending birth and recovery. Although the end result of a beautiful baby makes everything worthwhile, the complications experienced in pregnancy and the pain of childbirth or recovery from a Caesarean are not to be underestimated. You may be feeling nervous as you contemplate the final leg of your journey through pregnancy into parenthood.

Giving birth, despite being a natural process, can have a huge effect on a new mum, both physically and emotionally. It is dramatic, far from painless, and exhausting, with even the wealth of joyful emotions leaving you feeling wrung out. You may find that your experience takes an unexpected turn, even if the birth is straightforward.

Remembering your 'goal' and the amazing thing you are doing by carrying your baby can help in the most painful, frustrating times as you endure the discomforts of pregnancy. Although I knew I had to have a Caesarean and could prepare, to a degree, both practically and emotionally for the birth, I could not have known that I would experience complications with my scar and that it would be a slow, painful road to full healing.

God is with us in every moment of life. He wants to bear our pain and bring us through suffering, surrounding us with his peace and comfort. Take some time to reflect on the love that makes it possible to go through great pain. Verses of scripture on pain and suffering can be challenging; certainly, being 'patient in affliction' is no small task and perseverance isn't easy. Bring to God those things in your life that cause you distress, pain or discomfort. Acknowledge before him that, in times of trial, being joyful is far from our natural response, and to persevere requires God's grace and strength when ours is fading. Take your pain and upset feeling before God in prayer, and relinquish the struggle into the loving arms of the one who can strengthen and build your character through endurance. Seek him afresh for the courage to stand once more and keep going towards the finishing line.

BIBLE VERSES
Hebrews 12:1 and Romans 5:3–4

Dear Lord, thank you that, whatever pain or discomfort I experience in my life, your love and your word are there to comfort and uphold me when I turn to you. However hard the road of suffering, give me the strength to focus on the goal of carrying my child safely into the world and to remember that the outcome will be worth every temporary pain. I pray that I would experience a fresh sense of your presence beside me each step of the way. May I find joy in the midst of pain and seek your strength when perseverance feels impossible, taking heart from the knowledge that you are my hope and strength. Amen

Mummy guilt

Feelings of responsibility about the choices you make for your child begin long before they are born, and guilt that you could not possibly have anticipated suddenly pervades your thinking. This strong sensation, often termed 'mummy guilt', can be surprising in its intensity and continues in many variations, through pregnancy and into parenthood. Worries about what you've eaten, your ability (or inability) to be a parent, and many other anxieties flood your mind as you seek to do the best for your child, from the moment you know of their existence.

These anxieties only magnify and multiply, given the chance, once your baby arrives. You might feel guilty about anything from your feeding choices to your feelings about motherhood, and there will be times when you get grumpy or feel as if you are a huge failure as a parent. I was astonished by the power of this hitherto unknown emotion, and I lost count of the times I said to my husband, 'I feel bad, because…'. This sentence could end with any number of logical or illogical feelings of guilt and self-deprecation.

Feelings of failure or self-criticism, with the guilt that they induce, are very real, yet they often arise simply from our own unrealistic expectations. No amount of reassurance erases these feelings, so visceral is the strength of emotion about one's child, but be encouraged that the shortcomings that make you feel so terrible are, in all likelihood, not as huge as they seem. They probably matter so greatly only to you. Believe people when they tell you, 'It's OK, you're doing your best!'

When we feel that we fall short and don't measure up, God wants to reassure us and take away our guilt. Take some time to bring your feelings of unworthiness, failure and guilt to him. Reflect upon the things you know you have genuinely done wrong in all areas of your life, but be kind to yourself and accept that many of the faults that you dwell upon are not as bad as you perceive them to be. Know that God can take away all our guilt, so, however inadequate you feel, you *are* good enough. Jesus died so that we could live in freedom. He surrendered his guiltless person so that we could relinquish every anxiety and know true forgiveness. You may need to remind yourself of this truth time and again, as you continue your walk with God and your journey into parenthood.

BIBLE VERSES
Romans 8:1–2 and Acts 13:38–39

Dear Lord, thank you that I can know forgiveness and freedom when I bring my guilt and worry to you. You know my every anxiety, the things I feel I lack and my innermost insecurities. Forgive me when I fall short; help me to discern those failings for which I need to ask your forgiveness and those actions and feelings for which I am condemning myself unnecessarily. Help me to weigh my thoughts and commit them to you. Take my feelings of shame and inadequacy and fill my mind instead with the knowledge that I am accepted and loved, set free by Christ. Amen

------ *Making room* ------

The final countdown on your pregnancy is underway, or perhaps your road through the adoption or fostering process is nearing its end. Very soon, now, you will be getting your home prepared to welcome your new arrival, ready for the moment when your baby starts the journey into parenthood with you. As the impending changes to your daily life start to become a reality, you begin to think of the ways your life and home will be transformed. With the arrival of your child, there will be a huge restructuring of your usual routine and your lifestyle will shift dramatically to accommodate it.

Preparing to welcome your baby into the family home involves much joy but also some massive practical and emotional adjustments. On this final stage of your journey, you will be anticipating the upheaval that is to come and the way your family dynamics will change. Take some time to talk with your partner and family about the way things might be different, and how making room for a new, all-consuming tiny person will change the way you operate in your daily life.

I remember the great excitement of this final countdown, the realisation that very soon we would start afresh with our newborn. Slightly apprehensive about the imminent alteration to life as we knew it, we chatted frequently about what it might be like to have our baby actually here at last. Making ready your home and heart is thrilling, yet disorientating. It was wonderful to prepare the nursery, Moses basket and all the little things our baby would need. However, a new baby will, in reality, take over most of the rooms in your house, not just the allocated nursery. It will stretch your capacity to think of others, so balancing the demands of this small baby with your existing relationships will take time and understanding.

In our faith-life, we often forget to invite God not only to inhabit our heart but also to be a living presence in our home and family life. In practice, how often do we include him in our daily routine and relationships? Do you give God 'house room'? Be honest about the ways you might need to make space in your life for God, asking him to be central in your family. Take some time, as you prepare to accommodate your baby, to reflect on whether you can also make room in your heart for God. Do you need to welcome him afresh into your family home and adjust your relationship with him too, as you welcome the baby?

```
BIBLE VERSE
Joshua 24:15
```

Father God, thank you that I am now making the last preparations to welcome a baby into my home and life, as my journey into parenthood reaches the final stage. Be with me as I get ready, as far as possible, emotionally and practically. Forgive me when I do not make room for you in my heart or make my relationship with you a priority in my life. Help me to bring to you my anxieties in this time of anticipation and to invite you to be central in my heart and home once more. Amen

_____

_____

_____

_____

_____

_____

_____

_____

God's plans, not our own

With the arrival of your baby fast approaching, your arrangements will be in place for when the moment finally comes. You will have made decisions about your preferences for the birth and will be thinking of all the ideal options for the care of your baby, or you may have finally completed the process of becoming a foster or adoptive parent. It is wonderful to make decisions and approach the impending journey of parenthood with a strategy. A reassuring plan of action helps to ease the nerves, both for you and for those who are preparing to support you with the birth or arrival and care of your baby.

However, like so many other times in life, the best laid plans sometimes have to change, by choice or necessity. Before the delivery of your baby, spend some moments considering how you might need to adapt your thinking. Talk to friends and family about their experiences if you can; very few new parents are able to stick to their original preferences to the letter. There is a strong chance that your birth plan, feeding ideals and perceptions of how life will be with your newborn will turn out to be drastically different from the way you imagined them during your pregnancy or as you prepared for parenthood. Medical complications, exhaustion and many other uncontrollable factors may mean that you have to make significant changes to the plan you had, in small or very big ways.

I was determined to breastfeed our second son, if I could, having fed our very hungry first son a combination of breastmilk and formula. However, our new baby required very regular feeds and blood sugar monitoring due to gestational diabetes. This meant that he had to have formula at intervals. Within days of his birth it became clear that it would be problematic to establish breastfeeding, despite my perseverance. It was a huge emotional struggle for me to accept that I had to relinquish my hopes and switch to bottle feeding, for my baby's health and my sanity. I certainly didn't make the change lightly and it took much reassurance from loved ones for me to find peace and move on.

It is not easy to bring our plans and hopes to God, in any area of our lives, only to find that his plan is nothing like our 'ideal'. Bring to God in prayer your hopes and plans for the birth and care of your baby, surrendering your desires and knowing that God has our lives in his hands and can comfort you when plans are forced to change. Ask that he might help you accept unforeseen alterations and give you the strength to trust in the path that he has set for you and your baby.

BIBLE VERSE
Jeremiah 29:11

Dear Lord, thank you that I can be secure in times when everything else is in a season of change, because your love for me is constant. May I seek your plans for my life as I prepare for the arrival of my child and the realisation that my plans may not come to fruition in the way that I envisaged. Give me the courage to face the unknown and the often rocky road of early parenthood and to place each part of the process under your watchful love. Amen

Section Two

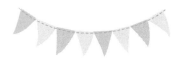

**PARENTHOOD
PRAYER JOURNEY**

------ *One moment at a time* ------

Your new role as a parent begins from the moment your little one is born or your child arrives. The enormity and complexity of this new chapter can be frightening, despite the feelings of relief and elation at your newborn's safe arrival. The implications of the many new skills and functions that a baby will need you to perform can come as a huge shock, especially as you are launched straight into the job. No one can fully prepare for this change to daily life.

When we became parents, the new routine felt daunting. In order to handle the weight of new responsibility, I made a conscious choice to take one job at a time, reminding myself to focus on that when I felt myself getting overwhelmed. Although it's great to establish a routine, thinking ahead even to the next day can be impossible at first, so we took it little by little, finding that each feed and nappy change, day and night, was different from the last. If this approach works for you, let go of the expectations that would normally be placed on you. Adopt a different pace. Allow space for you and your baby to adjust to this new life together, and get to know each other slowly.

There are times in our walk with God when we need to take life step by step and recognise the littlest of achievements, appreciating the worth in each small thing that we do for God and not looking too far along the road. The imagery of a lamp in Psalm 119:105 is helpful in this respect. God lights our path just far enough for us to see the next step, not the whole road. God's word, and the comfort of knowing he is with us, can light our way even when we struggle. Responsibilities can be all-consuming, especially with a newborn, so take each moment as it comes and commit each footstep to God in prayer.

BIBLE VERSES
Lamentations 3:21–23 and Psalm 119:105

Heavenly Father, knowing you are with me in each moment of the day and night with my baby is a great comfort. Help me to resist worrying about the road ahead and simply to trust that you will light my path as I take each new step into the unknown. Thank you that you go before me, knowing my needs and those of my baby. Give me the strength I need to take one moment at a time, as I adjust to a new path that is different each day. I praise you for the joy in the little moments of the day and night as my baby and I get to know each other and learn together. Help me to cherish this time of not rushing, and to find peace in your presence. Amen

------ Transformed perspectives ------

The journey into parenthood and the beginning of this new role bring many changes, some of seismic proportions. There are some big alterations to be made in your daily life and relationships now that your little one has arrived. However relaxed you try to be, the introduction of a new baby into your life will bring significant changes to your perspective on the world, your relationship with others and God.

Change at any stage of life is an important experience. I remember the huge impact on our home life as we adjusted to the all-consuming presence of this tiny person who now shared our home. We had to make an effort to find ourselves as a couple in the midst of the upheaval, but there was also a great sense that we were being brought closer together as we navigated an uncharted sea of emotions. I also found that becoming a mummy gave me a change of perspective on my relationship with other women, particularly with my own mum, as we now shared the experiences of motherhood.

Reflect on the ways in which becoming a parent has changed your perspectives. Spend some time focusing on God, fixing your gaze upon him as a constant, loving presence in times of adjustment. Be gentle with yourself as you bring before God your honest feelings about the physical and emotional changes you are experiencing and the impact they are having on you.

Consider how knowing God in your life has altered your perspective in other ways, before you became a parent. How might he be changing the way you see things now? Trust that God is with you and at work in you at this time. Invite him to renew your outlook and ask him for the strength to face the difficult parts of this adjustment to a different life. Becoming a parent not only brings a new relationship with a rather demanding little personality, but it also has an impact on other close relationships with family and friends. Take time to seek God's guidance in all of these changes.

BIBLE VERSE
Romans 12:2

Dear Lord, thank you that you are with me in this time of adjustment and that you are interested in every part of my life and relationships. Help me to trust that you are renewing me from within, however bewildered I feel. Transformation can be hard! Help me to process all the changes and to seek you as I embrace this new role, with its huge physical and emotional impact. I pray that you would guide me and those who share this journey with me as we are faced with new perspectives. Help us to find ways to accommodate the inevitable adjustments in our relationship. Help me to remember the transforming power of your love. I invite you to renew my mind and keep me grounded in you, in the midst of changes. Amen

------ *Absolute reliance* ------

Children have an unquestioning trust in their parents from the moment they are born. They look to you for reassurance, to know that they are secure and loved. It is natural for them to trust you completely and rely on you entirely for everything. This can feel like a frightening prospect to you—a huge responsibility that will last a lifetime. However, you are not alone in feeling the enormity of the task ahead as you begin the journey of parenting a newborn. Your new role, despite being disorientating and scary, is an amazing privilege and a gift from God as he entrusts your child or children into your loving care. Your child will continue to need your help in many ways through all stages of life. Even as they grow in independence and are no longer helpless and reliant on you for every need, they will still turn to you as their parent in times of trouble, worry or great joy.

Since we had very little experience with babies before becoming parents, the responsibility of caring for a small person who was so utterly reliant upon us meant that we had to learn very quickly. I often prayed, as I tried to fathom what my baby needed at any given time, 'Lord, help him to let me know if he needs something, and help me to know what to do.' I still pray this prayer most nights as I put my three-year-old to bed.

My child's trust in my parental care for his needs continues, despite his growing independence, and I in turn rely on my heavenly Father to help me in the parenting role. Do you daily put your trust in your heavenly Father, in the same way that your baby unwaveringly trusts you? Do you realise that he wants to provide for every need and wants you to rely on him absolutely? Perhaps, as you have grown in faith, you have begun to bring your needs to God less often, becoming more independent. Reflect on ways you could trust God more implicitly, and the areas of life that you need to surrender into his loving care. Consider those times when you've relied on him in the past and taken every little anxiety to him in prayer. Perhaps you need to admit to those aspects of life that make you feel as helpless as a small baby, and allow God to be your strength and guide.

BIBLE VERSES
Proverbs 3:5–6

Father God, thank you for entrusting this child into my care. Help me to reassure, comfort and provide for my baby, who places unquestioning trust in me. Lord, be a close and comforting presence, especially when the responsibility feels overwhelming. Help me to rely on you as my heavenly Father and trust you as your child. Forgive me when I fail to seek you with the needs of my day. May I remember that you are with me in every part of caring for my baby and may I look to you for guidance. Help me to place my confidence in you implicitly, in all areas of my own life. Amen

Future in their eyes

Looking into their eyes, you can't help wondering what your baby will look like in the future. Already, within this child is the potential for all they will grow up to be. This is an awesome thing to reflect on, as you look at such a tiny person, lying quietly looking back at you. It's monumental to wonder what kind of personality this new creation will develop. I remember looking at our newborn baby and wondering what his voice would sound like when he talked. What would his future hold? What kind of work would those little hands do, as yet so delicate that I was nervous even to trim the nails?

You may have some long-held hopes for what your child might achieve or the life you want them to experience. Dream big dreams for your baby! Believe that this child has the potential to live an amazing life, but remember that you will need to accept and love them even more fiercely if they don't achieve their goals or if they choose paths that you would have preferred them to avoid. Reflect on the sort of things you hope for. Bring to God these hopes and any fears for the future, as you see your baby beginning to grow and change already.

God sees in you, his child, all the possibilities for your future achievements. He knew you before you knew him, and he knows the paths set before you and your child. You may feel that you are not the person you could be, or that hopes and dreams you held for yourself while you were growing up have not been realised. Accept that you have limitations but believe that God can help you develop and change, through his grace, forgiveness and love. He knows all the potential within you, and he created you for a purpose.

BIBLE VERSE
Psalm 139:16

Dear Lord, thank you that as I hold my child, I hold a life filled with huge potential. It's incredible to think that this baby will grow and change into an adult with their own voice, skills and place to inhabit within the world. Thank you that you give each of us a unique and important role to play and that you know our full capacity.

Help me to support and guide my child as they grow. May I encourage them to discover their gifts and abilities, celebrating their personal achievements. Help me to remember that I too have been created for a reason; you have given me all the skills I need to fulfil my role in your plan. May I seek your guidance when I feel that my dreams have remained dormant or when they seem unachievable. I pray that you grant me the courage and faith I need to pursue opportunities for growth, and to know that, with your grace and forgiveness, it is never too late to become the person you designed me to be. Amen

Made in the image of…

When your child is born, there may be a striking resemblance to a parent or other family member. Perhaps you can see a fascinating mixture of recognisable features, going together to make up an amazing and unique brand new person. From the moment you or others see your baby, or when the photos are passed round, there will be a range of comments, speculation and assertions about who your newborn looks like. With both my sons, we spotted a distinct resemblance to their father and paternal grandfather as soon as we laid eyes on them. Comments like 'He's the image of his father!' were regularly heard, although both boys also have some of my features and our elder son has grown to resemble me more as a toddler. It is intriguing to see how a baby's appearance alters over a short time from birth and then as the months and years go by. You may not notice the changes as much as other people do because you are with your children daily, but looking back over photos can bring some surprises.

The Bible describes how humankind was created in God's image. How does this knowledge inspire you to reflect his characteristics in the world in which you live? Do we present the image of God to the people we meet? Would they recognise our heavenly Father in our appearance? Take some time to think about the image you present to the people you encounter in the world.

BIBLE VERSE
2 Corinthians 3:18

Father God, thank you that you created each of us in your image, that we might resemble you in our actions and be a reflection of your love in the world. I give you praise for the wonderful little being that I hold in my arms, the tiny person who is utterly new and unique, yet has inherited distinguishable family features. Forgive me when I fall far short of your image, my heavenly Father, in my words and actions. Help me to seek you and to strive to live a life that demonstrates your love to the people I encounter. Amen

The best person for the job

You may be feeling terribly unprepared and not at all expert as a parent. In truth, all new parents have to learn as they go along, however easy they make it look. Be assured, you are the best person for this job and you were chosen by God to parent your child. Regardless of how many books, websites and blogs you avidly consulted on parenting and baby development stages, you can't fully anticipate the challenges you will face as you get accustomed to being a parent for the first time. It is a huge learning process for you and your baby. There are no 'right' answers every time; no amount of study or research will prevent you from failing at times. However, through experience, as you deal with the occurrences that are particular to you and your family, you will also learn more than you thought possible with your baby.

This is not to say that the reassurance and advice provided by books and websites are not valuable; they can certainly make a huge difference, letting you know that others are going through the same adjustments and confusion. I found that speaking to other new parents and reading blogs on the highs and lows of parenting provided much-needed validation. I felt reassured that I was doing OK and that everyone finds it difficult and perplexing as they navigate the early days with a newborn. Even as a novice parent, only you can fulfil the particular purpose God has for your life, and he has given you the gifts and skills to fulfil each part. It's OK to 'fail' and get it wrong in testing times. Take some time to reflect on all that you have learnt and achieved as a new parent and give yourself credit for it, rather than focusing on the things you feel clueless about.

In our walk with God, he never condemns us when we get things wrong or have to repeat the same learning experience over and over again. Do you need to seek guidance from God, humbly asking for his grace as you make mistakes and learn? He is the best teacher and is walking beside you as you grow into an experienced parent and as you strive to learn and develop as a Christian. Seek his counsel and instruction as you adapt to this new task of parenthood.

BIBLE VERSE
Romans 12:6

Father God, during the learning process of new parenthood, may I remember to come to you, my teacher and counsellor. Help me to bring those times when I feel underqualified or unequal to the task and to trust that you would not give me more than I can handle. Thank you that, in my new relationship with my baby and in all areas of my life, you equip me with the gifts and strength I need to fulfil the tasks you set before me. Please help me to grow through experience and be encouraged daily as I develop new skills. Amen

When an inner strength
------ takes over ------

Often, when a baby arrives, the new mum can manage incredibly well, taking care of her tiny newborn from the very beginning, on little or no sleep. The hormones produced at this time, including adrenalin, can give you a natural capacity to do more than you thought possible. Despite the physical aftermath of the birth, something seems to keep you going in ways you couldn't possibly have done before.

In our shared exhaustion after the birth of our second son, my husband was surprised by how tired he felt, yet I seemed to just power through, even with night feeds. I had to reassure him (in his 'Daddy guilt') that I had the advantage of the hormones helping me cope. His support of me, sharing the care of our toddler and newborn as well as going out to work, meant that he was bound to be physically and emotionally drained.

Even if you feel quite the opposite to empowered and resilient, God is with you through every peak or trough of energy. His Holy Spirit can minister to us in all our most testing and bewildering moments of life. God's strength is at work most powerfully in our times of weakness and need. In this time of emotional turmoil, it is likely that you will feel extremely happy then utterly incapable by turns, as your hormones continue to fluctuate. This is very normal, but do not be afraid to seek support if you feel that you are not settling down and emotions of despair or anxiety are not tempered by times of joy. Share your feelings with the people close to you and perhaps ask them to pray with you as you draw near to the God of the impossible and ask again for his guidance on the journey through early parenthood.

Call to mind those instances in your walk with God when you have felt something take over—a peace or vitality that could not be explained by your own human capacity. This was his Holy Spirit at work, enabling you to do more than you imagined possible. Perhaps there have been times in your life when you've overcome seemingly insurmountable difficulties and have known God's strength and the power of his Holy Spirit upholding you. Give thanks for these times and ask God to give you a fresh knowledge and experience of his strength and grace in the midst of all the newness of parenthood.

> **BIBLE VERSES**
> **Ephesians 3:16–20**

Lord God, thank you that I can find my strength in you and be renewed by the power of your Holy Spirit. Help me to seek a fresh experience of the peace and fortitude that come from drawing near to you in my weakness, relying on your power and grace. May I know when to ask for help from others, and may I be gentle with myself whether I am elated or overwrought. I bring all these emotions to you. Amen

Finding God in the
------ messy and mundane ------

Taking time to meet with God among the daily messy jobs of parenting can be both difficult and insightful. Some of the more mundane and repetitive tasks of parenthood can be unpleasant and unrelenting, such as changing nappies or trying to keep up with the inevitable increase in laundry. I found a curious kind of inspiration as I reflected while dealing with the not-so-sweet side of my darling baby's care. With the time to think, as I repeatedly changed nappies or put yet another load of washing on, I met with God in new ways. God is an expert at dealing with mess and confusion, and I was able to reflect on this aspect of his character as I worked.

The more monotonous parts of looking after your newborn's needs can be arduous and boring, and it's OK to admit it. Try to see, through it all, the bigger picture of the amazing task of raising a child. God is interested in every part of our daily life, and he wants us to invite him to be with us in the midst of the mess and chaos. Bring to God your frustrations as you repeat the tedious everyday routines. Talk to God as you fold piles of laundry or do the washing-up. You might bring to him the things in your life that need 'cleaning', asking for a fresh start.

In the busy, tiring whirl of new parenthood, with a demanding baby, the idea of finding 'quiet' time for yourself with God can be laughable. You might find that you have lost the time or enthusiasm to read the Bible or settle into quiet prayer. Reflect on ways to give time to God in your new routine, perhaps during the night feeds or by downloading a daily Bible verse app on your phone. Often, as new parents, our prayers are sent in bursts of requests or as 'arrow prayers'—short heartfelt cries to God. Ask God to help you bring your prayers to him as and when you can. Don't underestimate the might behind those short, earnest prayers. Prayer 'on the go' may feel less significant than the lengthy quiet times you previously enjoyed. However, by talking to God in these snatched moments, you are including him in a real, personal way in every part of your life. In some ways, this may be a more meaningful form of worship than eloquently worded prayers.

87

> **BIBLE VERSES**
> **Zephaniah 3:17 and Deuteronomy 31:8**

Dear God, thank you that you are with me in every little task as I care for my baby. Help me to find new ways to meet with you, to share my daily life with you and to bring you my prayers. When my day feels humdrum and tedious, may I find encouragement in knowing that I am doing something important, tending to my baby's needs and comfort. Forgive me when I feel frustrated by these ordinary tasks, and help me to see reflections of you at work in these moments. Amen

Washed clean

Bathing your newborn can be a nerve-wracking experience at first. Carefully holding and gently cleaning that tiny person is a really special part of learning to care for your baby. However beautiful your little one is, you will have discovered from the day they arrived that they do not stay clean for long after emerging from the bath smelling so very sweet. Also, they don't always enjoy the experience. When we first bathed our new baby at home, he objected noisily. As it was November, he preferred being cosy in his Babygro. Our second son was born in June and has loved water from birth. It is a real delight that they now love having splashy bath-time fun together.

I find that water helps me reflect and connect with God, whether I'm swimming or just taking a shower. I often pray at these times and feel very inspired and 'alive' in water, the source of vitality. There are many biblical references to water and cleansing, from the waters of baptism to the imagery of the water of life that Jesus offers, or of being washed clean by the blood of Jesus. When we bring all that is messy and unpleasant in our life to God, with a true heart of repentance, we are purified, washed clean of all our sin and shame by the redeeming blood of Jesus.

Whenever you bath your baby, take a bath or shower yourself, or drink water, spend some time reflecting on the symbolism of water in your faith journey. Give thanks to God for the blessing of clean water to wash in and drink. Perhaps call to mind your baptism or a time when you felt significantly restored and revitalised in your faith-life. Bring before God in prayer those areas of your life where you need to be refreshed again now. Lay before him the places where you feel spiritually 'thirsty' or need to ask for forgiveness. Know that he can wash you clean, and remember once more the redemptive grace poured out for you upon the cross.

> **BIBLE VERSES**
> **1 John 1:9 and John 4:7–15**

Dear Lord, thank you that I can cleanse my baby in the bath, after even the most messy of times. I praise you for the blessing of clean, refreshing water and the wonderful smell of a freshly bathed baby. Forgive me when I do not bring my own mess and transgressions to you, the source of all forgiveness, purity and love. Help me to draw strength and refreshment from the spring of eternal life. May I make a new start and be washed clean as I seek you, the font of renewal and grace. Amen

Held in his hands

How amazing it is to see the tiny hands of your newborn—delicate and fragile, yet strong enough to grasp your finger tightly from the first moments of life. It is fascinating to look at their hands compared to yours, so small, with those minute nails. This tiny version of a person has such potential to grow from helpless babe to an adult who is able to use their hands to do so many things.

The imagery of hands and being held resonates strongly with me. When I looked at my baby's tiny hands, I marvelled at the thought of how those hands would grow to hold a spoon, create art and give hugs. It led me to reflect upon God's mighty hands, which placed the stars into space, yet gently hold me, his child. I was a very premature baby, born three months early, and my mum tells how she could do nothing at the time but prayerfully place me in God's hands each night. I continue to place myself in his hands as an adult, and I pray the same prayer for my children. Praying for your baby as you hold them or watch over them while they sleep, or when they are ill, is very powerful. Committing them into God's care and praying with them as they grow is a huge blessing and reassurance.

Do you place yourself into the loving hands of God, your heavenly Father? Just as a baby can exert a tight grip on your finger or hair, we can hold firmly on to the hand of God. He holds us tightly in his hands and doesn't let go, however old we grow. The hands that created the universe are wide and comforting, yet able to hold you safe as a tiny child. You can find rest, knowing that you are secure in his hands, just as your child places their tiny hand in yours.

BIBLE VERSES
John 10:28–29

Heavenly Father, those minuscule hands reaching out to me, the parent, are a wonder of your creation. Thank you for my child, their hands and feet and every detail that is so precious and unique. I give you thanks and praise you for the blessing of holding my baby and the privilege of seeing this tiny form grow and develop. I place myself once again into your care and ask that you would comfort and hold me tight as a child of God, living my life safe in your hands. Amen

The shower 'window'

It is really important, in the exhausting early days of parenthood, to take time for yourself when a momentary 'window' becomes available. Without guilt, allow yourself the space for a shower, a nap or a moment of reflection, perhaps when your baby is sleeping or being minded by someone else. Your natural tendency, when you get a brief gap in your day, will be to use the time in a productive way, to cook, clean or organise laundry. Of course, if these things help you feel better, you can do them. However, choosing to take a few minutes to yourself is not selfish or irresponsible. You need time to relax. Stop for a moment. Sleep, pray, drink warm tea, read a magazine, play music—do something, even just for a short while. Whatever other mums seem to be doing with their time, there are no prizes for trying to be a superhero and ending up strung out or in a physical and emotional heap. This will not help you or your baby.

I learnt quite quickly that this 'shower window' is a most precious interval in the busy new routine. I found that if I raced around doing all kinds of useful things in the house, I would miss the chance to get a shower before my baby woke again for a feed. I also realised that it was fun for him to watch me from his bouncy chair as I cooked, washed up or folded laundry, and chatted about what I was doing.

Do you have the right priorities in your spiritual life? Do you dash around doing so many things for others that you neglect to rest in God, taking time to talk to him, read a little of his encouraging word or wait upon him? Consider those activities that fill your life. Where could you make God part of your busy day? Let go of any feelings of guilt over the tasks not yet done, and allow yourself some space just to be. Breathe. Find tranquillity and replenishment through prayer. Do something that makes you happy. Relax and know that time spent in restful contemplation is not laziness. Ask God to ease your mind and body as you rest prayerfully, for just a little while, in his presence.

BIBLE VERSES
Matthew 11:28–30

Lord God, I thank you that even within a hectic and packed schedule of 'doing' as I care for my baby, there are moments of respite to be found and used wisely, to revive my weary body and to help me meet with you. Help me to discern which tasks are urgent and which can wait a short while, to allow me a much-needed break from activity and the chance to rest in you. May I seek your peace and know that I can allow myself time to renew my strength for the responsibilities of home and family life. Help me not to neglect myself or you, and to find a happy balance between fulfilling these roles and finding a place of solitude where I can encounter you. Amen

I've got you!

Sometimes, you may be at a loss about how to soothe your crying baby, having tried all the obvious solutions—food, nappy change, winding. Then you realise that all your newborn really wants is for you to hold them close, as reassurance that they are secure and loved. I have often found myself simply walking around, holding my baby tight and saying, 'I've got you' over and over to comfort him. At other times, my husband would feel a bit dejected, having tried everything to soothe him, when he calmed down almost instantly upon being handed to Mummy.

There are days when nothing but the most familiar smell and sound of Mummy will do. This can be hard for others who are trying their best to comfort your child. However, it is no reflection on others' ability to care for your baby, when you consider that the mother's heartbeat and voice were a constant soundtrack throughout pregnancy. Being held close can still be the best form of comfort when all other needs have been met. This is particularly true in the early days or nights, after your baby has been so rudely evicted from the warmth and security of the womb, where the constant swishing sounds and the familiar rhythm of your heartbeat were all they knew. They simply want to be near to that familiar heartbeat, to rest and feel secure in your arms.

In your life and your journey of faith, do you need to hear again from God and to believe that he says to you, as his child, 'I've got you'? Sometimes no practical action, clever words or deep scriptural revelations are required; we simply want and need to draw near to the heart of God, to know that he is holding us tight and everything is in his control. We can rest like a child and know that he is cradling us in his arms.

BIBLE VERSES
Psalm 62:5–7 and 91:1–5

Father God, help me to know when to stop searching for solutions and simply rest in your arms. Help me to come again into your embrace, to ask for the comfort that only you can bring, and to know your heart for me as I find my security in you. Forgive me when I try so hard to discover a reason or solve a problem, and get so caught up in trying fruitlessly to fix something, that I forget to ask you to hold me. Help me to remember that you have got me safe. I pray that I might discover afresh the peace and joy of knowing that you hold me and my child in your care. Amen

------ *Bedtime routine, take 3* ------

There are days when the repetition of nappy and clothing changes seems endless. It can be frustrating and exhausting when you finally reach bedtime and get your baby snuggly, only to find that they need yet another full change within moments, and are then sick over the fresh outfit. I remember finding it incredible that my sweet little baby boy could remain in one set of clothes for most of the day, yet produce a marvellously messy 'hat trick' of bodily functions around his bedtime feed in his dimly lit nursery. It always seemed to happen when I was least expecting it or when I was most tired. Of course, nappy dramas and frequent clothing swaps are expected with a newborn but there are times when the sequence of events is almost funny. Your angelic little one can increase your washing pile considerably, in a matter of minutes, with their startling capacity to explode from either end, or both.

If we are honest, as Christians, we can go through a similar process in our life and faith, making the same bad choices again and again. We often do not learn from our mistakes but keep on getting in a mess. Do you repeat the same wrong actions in your life? Are there patterns of behaviour that you know you need to change? Despite your resolve, do you find yourself always saying or doing the thing that you know isn't right or kind?

Lay these mistakes before the Lord, admitting that you need help in breaking your patterns of behaviour. Be honest with yourself and God, but take heart as you determine to make efforts to change. God can give you a fresh start and a clean slate, with the mess and wrongdoings forgotten. Walk confidently as you continue your journey of faith, striving to grow through your lapses in judgement, in the knowledge that God's grace makes you free indeed.

BIBLE VERSES
Psalm 103:12 and Isaiah 43:18–19

Dear God, thank you that even if I make the same mistakes repeatedly, you welcome me with forgiveness and a new start when I bring my transgressions to you. Forgive me when I do not learn but yet again find myself duplicating behaviour or words that I know are damaging to others or do not glorify you. Help me to forgive myself when I keep failing, believing that you accept my heartfelt repentance. Amen

_____

_____

_____

_____

_____

_____

_____

_____

_____

Grounded for a reason
------ and a season ------

The change in your lifestyle on becoming a parent can mean a sizeable adjustment. Your world becomes considerably smaller to begin with, and it is easy to feel isolated, as if you exist in a baby-focused microcosm. You might previously have been heavily involved in ministry activities at your church or had a busy social life, but now your days and nights are concentrated entirely upon your baby.

This can be a frustrating—or liberating—time of acclimatising to new parenthood. When you have settled into your new role, you may start to see new horizons. The prospect of attending mother-and-baby groups or having other new mums round for a coffee can be a real pleasure as you all enjoy this time with your small babies. It is also a season when you are able to be more available to support others. In the doctor's waiting room one day, when I met a woman from church who was experiencing a tough time, I invited her to come straight round to my home. Previously, in all likelihood, we would have had just a brief chat before I had to rush off to the next item on my day's agenda. You can bless others with your time. Becoming part of a whole different social scene, taking your baby to organised groups, out for walks or to church, opens up doors to minister and grow as you develop new ways of interacting with others. You will notice that you have conversations with strangers and friends that would never have taken place previously. Sharing the experiences of parenthood can be an amazing way to find firm friendships as you live out your faith.

Reflect on the way God can use you in your new environments. How could you support others, with empathy and compassion, in the busy world of mother-and-baby groups? Ask God to help you discern those people who might be lonely or struggling. Think of the people you could bless with a word of encouragement or a smile as you play with your babies in a group or pass each other in the supermarket in a fog of exhaustion. Do not underestimate the role you can play while you're 'grounded'. Parenthood can open up a very important ministry to others, as well as to the child you are raising. You can be a light for God at home with your baby or in the world where you now find yourself.

BIBLE VERSES
Matthew 5:14–16

Dear Lord, thank you that you are with me in this season of being 'grounded', when the usual commitments in my daily life are relinquished and I prioritise the needs of my new baby. Help me to find ways to cope with the different pace of life and not to feel isolated or useless. May I remember the huge ministry role that parenthood can bring. Help me to see it as a season of opportunity in which I can do new things as I seek to shine for you. Amen

------ *With you in the storm* ------

The changes and challenges of early parenthood can be stormy, turbulent and testing. You can feel blindsided by the emotional and physical turmoil. Although this is a season of great joy, it is mixed with times when you feel at a complete loss, disorientated by the constant onslaught of new responsibilities. It can leave you unsure of your ability to manage the enormous difference in your situation.

There were instances in the very early days and nights with our first baby when I was hit by sudden waves of doubt, anxiety and panic. Was I up to the task? It can be scary to think that this tiny helpless being is relying on you for every need. I clearly remember sobbing, for a few brief moments, every evening for the first three or four nights after I came home from hospital. These tears were as much an expression of happiness as they were an outpouring of the build-up of anxious emotions and anticipation. Although the feelings were fleeting, interspersed with crashing deluges of utter amazement and joy, they were a very real part of the emotional turbulence of the voyage of parenthood. You will be used to hormonal fluctuations and their effects, but nothing prepares you for the disconcerting blend of elation and panic that you feel by turns, as your body and mind are subject to a continuing flux of chemical transformations, until well after your baby's birth.

When these swells of emotion roll in, remember that God is right in the centre of the storm with you, guiding you through. Not only can he calm the raging waters but he is in the midst of the storm, holding you up and keeping you safe as you go through the waves. God's loving presence is available as an anchor that holds firm in the roughest seas. Reach out to him; cling to his promises when you feel you're barely keeping your head above water. Take time to reflect afresh on his strength, which is your firm foundation even when you feel far away from him and 'all at sea'. God is right there, his hand outstretched, guiding you and preparing you to walk upon the waters that threaten to engulf you. Do not be afraid to seek support if these overwhelming waves of emotion do not subside, but rest secure that, in time, all storms pass and calmer seas will follow.

> **BIBLE VERSES**
> **Isaiah 41:10 and Psalm 107:28–31**

Father God, in the moments when I feel overcome by the waves of emotion, help me to remember that you are near. You are my comfort and my place of safety; you give me strength when I need buoying up. Help me to cling to you, knowing that your love is steadfast even when everything I know seems to be shifting. Give me the courage to seek help when I need it, knowing that you can calm every fear. I stand once more upon your promises, my rock and my redeemer. Amen

_____

_____

_____

_____

_____

_____

_____

_____

------ *Take me with you* ------

Your baby wants to experience everything with you. The world is filled with new and exciting sights and sounds. Try telling your baby about the things in your garden or street as you stand looking out of the window together; talk to them about what you are doing in the bathroom or kitchen, or sing them a song. Babies delight in being with you, whatever you are doing.

With their developing awareness of their surroundings, babies also reach a stage when they experience separation anxiety. This is a strong emotion, as they are struck by a sense of very real fear that you have left them when you are out of view. Of course, they gradually learn that you always come back and no longer react so strongly each time. Our younger son has just reached this stage of development. He will cry with utter panic when I leave the room momentarily, but greets me with a beaming smile the moment I reappear, no longer concerned that I have (as I jokingly put it with both my babies) 'gone to the moon'.

There are times during this wobbly stage when you may have to carry your baby around the house with you on errands or to the bathroom. This can be quite wearing for you, but it does pass, and there can be great joy in it for both of you when you share every little experience with your baby. Rather than seeing it as a bind, enjoy the experience if you can. Your baby will soon be independent and exploring happily without needing to be in your arms constantly.

Reflect on how God wants us to acknowledge him with us through our day. He longs for us to invite him to be present, sharing in all we do. In times of anxiety, as we face the prospect of going into a scary situation, God's word reminds us that he will never leave us or forsake us. Consider ways in which you can make a deliberate effort to take God into each day's activities. Perhaps copy out the words of one of the Bible verses below and leave them where you will see them often. Pause before each important activity to pray, inviting God to go before you. Know that the God of comfort walks every path alongside you and is an ever-present source of courage and strength for the day.

```
BIBLE VERSES
Joshua 1:9 and Deuteronomy 31:6
```

Ever-present Lord, thank you that you want to accompany me everywhere I go, so that you experience the world with me. Help me to know that you go before me into each new day and walk beside me through everything I encounter. Give me the courage to make a deliberate effort to include you in my daily life. Forgive me when I do not share my fears or joys with you. May I remember that you can supply the courage and strength I need. I have only to seek your presence, with me at every step. Amen

------ Too tired to talk ------

Sheer exhaustion can mean you feel barely able to speak at times. Even the most talkative person can be floored when adjusting to life with a baby. With the all-consuming demands of your little one and the loss of any consistent sleep pattern, even if you used to chatter endlessly you may often find yourself sounding incoherent now.

Reflect on the opportunities that can be found when we stop talking and listen. The old adage that when we close our mouth we can more easily open our ears to hear is true when it comes to seeking God and hearing from him. When we are in a daze of fatigue, simply taking time to rest, giving our weary souls a moment of peace, can also allow us to open our hearts to God, giving him a chance to speak to us. I remember being dazed with exhaustion, awake in the night with a poorly baby or waiting for him to settle to sleep after a feed. I was unable to do more than sit in God's presence and allow his Spirit to wash over my anxiety. Yet it was in some of my weariest moments that he spoke a simple word to me, like 'I know' or 'Let it go'.

When you feel too tired to form words to pray, give God the chance to minister to you. Remain open to knowing his will, hearing from him and receiving the strength and grace he has for you, right in the middle of the longest night. When you are awake with your baby in the early morning, feeding, changing and comforting, the God who created you is also 'awake'. Invite him into these unearthly hours: God does not necessarily speak in audible words, but you may feel a sense of his presence, or a simple phrase or Bible verse will come to your mind as you listen. He may want to whisper gently, 'It's OK, I'm with you', just as you might say these words to your child in the watches of the night. Allow his Holy Spirit to minister to you, interceding for you when you are too tired even to utter a word of prayer.

BIBLE VERSES
Psalm 121 and Romans 8:26–27

Gentle Saviour, thank you that my soul can find rest in you even when I am the most tired. Help me to spend time listening to you in the quietness of the night or when I am too exhausted even to put my prayers into words. May your Holy Spirit refresh and guide me as I seek you. Help me to listen for your still, small voice and open my heart to hear from you. Thank you that you neither slumber nor sleep and that you are truly with me day and night. Help me to know the comfort of your loving presence in these times of exhaustion. Amen

Enjoy the moment

With the enormous demands of your parenting role, it is easy to forget to appreciate the present moment and take joy in little things. The endless cycle of feeding, changing and laundry is important, but sometimes you can let these chores wait for a while. Pause to reflect in the midst of all the activity, give your baby your full focus, and just 'be' for a few minutes. Sit and smile at the tiny miracle in front of you, and delight in the here and now. Babies grow quickly; as many parents will tell you, these days soon pass, so the washing-up can wait for a moment.

Since the day our first baby arrived, we have taken thousands of photographs of him and, later, his brother. These pictures are utterly precious, capturing so many treasured moments for us and our family and friends. However, do not lose the chance to participate in your baby's experiences while you try so hard to capture that perfectly timed photo. For example, I know from my own attempts that bubbles are notoriously tricky to capture on camera and it's often better simply to immerse yourself in the joy of chasing or watching them with your baby.

Sometimes we forget to stop and appreciate the importance of the present moment in our walk with God. We get so busy with everyday life, striving for the next goal, praying hard for a new job, house, relationship or opportunity in ministry, that we miss the blessings that God has for us in our current circumstances. Reflect on the unnoticed signs and wonders that God might be using to remind you to grasp the way he demonstrates his power and grace. Slow down and take time to appreciate the here and now, asking God to reveal his glory and help you to see that he is always working for your good, whatever your circumstances.

Looking back on your journey with God, think about those moments that seemed unimportant at the time, yet have played a significant part in your development and growth. Remember that, in life, in our parenting and in our faith journey, we often see in hindsight that the little things were among the most important.

BIBLE VERSES
Psalm 8:3–4

Dear Lord, thank you that you are with me in every moment of my life. You walk with me through the experiences of each day. Help me to remember that this time with my young baby will be short and precious, and to capture the memories created in the present moment. Forgive me when I get so concerned about the future, or impatient for answers to prayers for change, that I miss the joy and blessings in my present circumstances. Help me to trust you with the bigger picture and seek your grace in the smallest of instances. Amen

------ *Not alone on this path* ------

There can be an unfortunate tendency for parents to compete over their adored babies' progress and development. Whether deliberate or not, this competition makes new parents feel inadequate as they get to grips with the challenges their little blessing brings. As you journey through the myriad changes and new experiences, it can make a huge difference to share the trials and joys with other new parents, with whom you can talk honestly.

Misconceptions about how effortlessly others appear to adapt to this stage of life only serve to fuel your feelings of incompetence. We are often ashamed to admit when we are finding things difficult, but we are not the only ones struggling. Others are going through the same daily mix of amazement and bone-weariness and are also just trying to do the best for their baby. It is a huge comfort to receive reassurance from a good friend, realising that she can empathise because she is experiencing the same difficulties. When some close friends of ours had their two sons, shortly before us each time, we would regularly ask their advice and found it greatly heartening to share our journey into family life with them. We continue to spend time together in mutual support, friendship and fun times, benefiting from the wisdom of their experience.

In our Christian life, offering support to those who are newer to faith can be a huge blessing. Even if you are relatively young in your faith, you still have valid and useful experiences to share. Think about the people known to you who are at an even earlier stage of parenthood or faith development. Reflect on the ways you have grown in understanding and relationship with God since your faith was in its infancy. What did an older Christian say or do that made a positive difference to you? Ask God to give you opportunities to communicate with others who may need a word of encouragement as they navigate an earlier stage of their walk with the Lord.

BIBLE VERSES
Ecclesiastes 4:9–10

Dear God, in my journey as a new parent, thank you for those people you have placed in my life who have been through it all already and can offer advice and encouragement. Help me to seek someone to ask for guidance, if I do not yet have this kind of relationship with a fellow parent. Thank you, Lord, for those mentors who inspired and reassured me when my faith was new. I pray that you would open up conversations in which I can reassure and encourage younger Christians and make a difference in their journey of faith. Amen

----- *Everyone has an opinion* -----

When you begin your journey through parenthood, you are likely to be inundated with advice on all aspects of it from all manner of sources. Just as in any other part of your life, this advice is not always accurate or easy to accept, and is often given whether you asked for it or not. Advice can be reassuring and supportive, but it can also be unhelpful and confusing. You will quickly learn to laugh off a certain amount of the well-meaning but unwanted opinions that bombard you. Equally, you may well find that the helpful, practical suggestions of trusted friends, or your own parents, become a sought-after means of support and wisdom.

Some of the advice we received was contradictory to our own feelings, and we were adamant that we should make up our own minds about what was right for us, as our baby's parents. One of the most important things, as you share the care of your baby with your partner or others, is that you discuss and come to agreement on key points. In all the choices about how and what to feed your baby, what kind of nappies to buy, sleeping arrangements, the use of a dummy, discipline strategies and so many more issues, you must make decisions that you can agree on. Support each other in these choices, compromising where necessary to find the approach that suits your little family. It isn't always easy to stick to the agreed plan, but don't work at cross-purposes.

Reflect on times in your Christian life when you have been given really helpful, encouraging advice. Remembering those people who nurtured your faith, give thanks for wise counsel and the positive effect it has had on your continuing growth and maturing faith. Lift negative experiences of false teaching or misplaced zeal to the Lord, letting them go and choosing not to carry their effects any further. Consider those Christian friends or leaders whom you trust implicitly and respect for their wise and honest advice. If you do not currently have Christian friends or leaders whom you can ask for guidance, pray that God will bring the right person or group of people into your life, so that they might help you develop in faith. Remember that God and his word are the only infallible source of truth and guidance, although the supportive words and wise counsel of trusted friends are a gift from God.

BIBLE VERSES
James 3:17 and Proverbs 1:5

Dear Lord, thank you that you place into my life those who offer wisdom and guidance. Help me to forgive those who give unhelpful suggestions or are overly forceful in their opinions. Help me to decide with confidence how to raise my child, seeking your example and strength to know what is best. May I always seek you first, above all others, to guide and counsel me in all areas of my life. Amen

_____

_____

_____

_____

_____

_____

_____

_____

------ *Strong, passionate love* ------

It is impossible to comprehend the strength of feeling that you have towards your baby. You may have been astounded by how deeply you fell in love with the squishy little bundle that you carried safely through pregnancy and birth. You will have experienced other types of love in your life—the love you feel for your family, your partner or your closest friends—but your fierce love for your child is unlike any emotion you've felt before. However tough your journey into parenthood, your attachment to this new person is instinctive and can bowl you over. Perhaps you have endured an emotional journey to finally adopt or foster your child. You have seen many other people's babies before, yet yours captivated you entirely, even as you witnessed all the mess and pain that followed the moment of their birth.

The bonds of motherhood have grown and been strengthened throughout your pregnancy or steps to parenthood, and your love for this child was growing long before you met. The love of a parent for a child is all-consuming. You have the strongest of desires to protect and stand as an advocate for your child against the world.

Having wondered for many years whether I would ever have my own children, the overwhelming love I felt for our first son was huge. I remember being concerned when we were pregnant with our second baby, doubting whether I could love another child the way I loved my first. Yet the capacity to love did not divide when our second son arrived; it multiplied. My love for my precious littlest boy is just as deep and heartfelt, and the love I feel for my firstborn develops in new ways as I see him grow into boyhood, showing genuine tender love (most of the time!) for his baby brother.

God's love for us is without end; it does not falter when we waver in our faith or do the wrong thing. Like a parent's, his love is indescribably strong. He wants to protect and comfort you. God's love can encompass all his children. He feels so passionately about each of us that he came to earth in all the frailty of humanity, demonstrating the ultimate sacrificial love, to redeem us. God loved you with an unconditional love before you began your relationship with him, and even before you were born.

BIBLE VERSES
1 John 4:10 and John 3:16

Father God, the love I feel for my baby is incredible, powerful and overwhelming. Thank you that you love me with an unfailing love, the strength of which goes beyond human understanding. Help me to seek you, my heavenly Father, as I find my way along the parenting journey and experience a new kind of love for my child. Thank you that in your Son, Jesus, you embodied a love that overcame death and fear, so that I might know freedom. Amen

------ *Nothing lasts for ever* ------

When you are in a haze of sleepless nights and your days are filled with the constant repetition of feeds and nappy changes that all seem to merge together, remember that these times are not going to last for ever. Every stage of development that you go through with your baby is a temporary phase, however tough and long each day and night may feel right now. All too soon you will realise that the daily schedule has gradually changed and you will find yourself facing a whole new set of challenges.

With the passing of the weeks, then months, as your baby grows and develops, the range of baffling new experiences also changes. In this all-consuming series of things to learn and remember, it's easy to miss the many blessings that are scattered through each day. Babies grow quickly, so take time to enjoy the cuddles after a feed, the first smiles or your baby's amazement at light or different textures. Savour the precious moments among the tough ones. It can be hard to see the bigger picture when the days seem so arduous, yet, in the lifelong journey of parenthood, they are but fleeting moments. It will get easier and there can be joy in the middle of it all.

In our life of faith, we often see only the challenges we are currently facing, the things we feel we could do better, or our current disappointments. We fail to appreciate the tiny but significant changes that God is making in our lives or the blessings that he can reveal. Bring your weariness to God, praying that he might help you see these blessings on even the hardest days. Take refuge in the knowledge that God has given you strength to persevere through challenging times, and that everything lasts just for a season. God brings us to these times, and through them, for a reason. Our journey with God is not always plain sailing; it includes seasons of spiritual dryness, bad experiences or disappointments.

Bring before God your honest feelings when your experiences of parenthood or other aspects of life are not as you hoped or imagined. Take some time to read Psalm 18 and Ecclesiastes 3:1. If you find it helpful, reflect upon the reassuring words, that God is your refuge and strength. Cry out to him with praise or despair; he is with you in every season.

BIBLE VERSES
Ecclesiastes 3:1 and Psalm 18:1–2, 28

Dear Lord, thank you that you are my refuge, my shield and a constant presence in every changing season of my life. Be with me as I navigate all the new challenges of parenthood. May I find strength in knowing that whether the days are joyful or tough, none of these seasons lasts for ever, but your love is eternal. I bring to you my confusion and my hopes. Help me to remember the words of the psalmist and trust that 'you, Lord, keep my lamp burning; my God turns my darkness into light'. Amen

------ *Letting go and letting God* ------

It can be a significant emotional struggle to let others take care of your baby for you. Allowing family or friends to take over, even for a brief time, can be a wrench, particularly in the early days and weeks. Leaving the baby with someone you trust, even just to take a bath or get a much-needed nap, can lead to a bombardment of feelings, from guilt and worry to relief, then to more guilt for feeling relieved to get a break. However, it can be a healthy and necessary step, to give yourself time and to begin learning slowly to relinquish complete control, sharing the joys and responsibility of your new arrival with those who are more than willing to support you.

It is only natural to want to provide all the care and nurturing you possibly can give to your new arrival, but I remember realising that I also needed, even in small ways, to allow other people to help. This is not only important for you as a new parent, but it gives other relatives the opportunity to bond with your baby. Although you may feel that you must take sole responsibility for every little need, there is great release and joy in letting go and letting others be involved.

Reflect on any areas of your life where you need to relinquish control and let God take over. Sometimes it can be a long process to decide what to let go and what to hold on to. Are there worries that you are trying to face by yourself rather than entrusting them to God? In all areas of your life, do you leave your anxieties and 'what ifs?' with him, or do you continually take them back and try and sort them out yourself, increasing your anxiety? Spend some time thinking of the worries that you fruitlessly hang on to. However small your concerns might feel, God wants you to place the burden of them in his hands. List them in prayer and let them go; let God be God. This is easier said than done, of course, and you will need to repeat the surrendering of your concerns often, in many aspects of your life and on your journey into parenthood.

BIBLE VERSES
Philippians 4:6–7

Dear Lord, letting go and letting others help to look after my child can be an emotional wrench. Help me to trust others and gradually relinquish some of the responsibility without guilt or fear, accepting offers of help and rest. I entrust my child and their health and well-being to you, Lord, and ask you to strengthen me to let go of worry or control. Help me to begin a daily habit of bringing my concerns to you and letting you be God over all my anxieties. Help me to leave them with you and know the freedom of walking in peace, knowing that you hold my worries in your care. Amen

Exactly where you are
------ meant to be ------

In your journey through early parenthood, there are countless times when there is nothing you can do but feed and comfort your baby, day and night. Whether the baby is ill, teething or simply not settling, you are exactly where you are meant to be. Nothing is more important in the here and now with your little one than looking after their needs, taking each moment as it comes.

Of course, this can be harder to accept and adjust to than it is to say. When plans are forced to change and your schedule has to be cleared, so that you are reduced to doing nothing but placating your baby, feelings of frustration, disappointment and even boredom or anger are natural. It can feel as if your day has been 'wasted' or 'ruined' when events have to be cancelled or postponed. You are left feeling tired and even guilty. However, there is no activity more important than caring for your baby, and you are doing a fantastic job!

I have lost count of the number of times when yet another minor illness or disturbed night meant we had to put aside all other plans. Often, though, you realise on these days that an enforced rest or pause in activity can be beneficial. Take time, next time your plans have to be shelved, to find God in the pauses of life. When everything has to stop, he is with you.

Take a moment to seek God as you hold your poorly baby or deal with the physical and emotional fallout of all that is involved in looking after them. Read Colossians 3:23–24 and be encouraged that in every little thing you do for your baby, you are serving God, right where you are. Draw strength from him as you fulfil this important task, in which patience and peace may not come naturally.

Are there other things in your daily life that cause feelings of frustration or impatience? Bring to God those aspects of life that feel 'paused'. Hard as it can be to accept, God sometimes deliberately limits us, temporarily, so that we can grow where we are planted. Prayers may seem to go unanswered but sometimes he is saying 'Wait' rather than 'No'. Trust that, in those times when progress seems slow or non-existent, God is at work and is preparing you for the next stage of life.

> **BIBLE VERSES**
> **Colossians 3:23–24**

Father God, when I face frustrating pauses in life, help me to seek your strength and wisdom. Help me to know that when I care for my baby, nothing else is more important and other activities can wait. Give me the grace I need to perform these tasks with all my heart, as I serve you in the role of motherhood. In times of frustration, when progress is halted, may I find rest, comfort and a sense of assurance that you are using these days to prepare me for your unfolding plan. Amen

------ Through the eyes of a child ------

Everything in the world is a wonder to a baby. Even from the earliest days of life, a newborn will respond to light and noises. Your baby's eyes slowly adjust after birth to focus on you and the people around them, gazing into the face that belongs to the familiar voice of Mummy.

In the early days, weeks and months, your baby will quickly develop a keen interest in the environment and will be inundated with new sensory encounters daily—hearing birdsong, seeing the sunlight filtering through tree branches, observing all the amazing sights and sounds of the world. When you see the joy on that tiny face, with the delight of each new experience, you cannot fail to be struck afresh by the wonders of the natural world. Your baby has so much to discover!

It was fascinating to see our firstborn focus his gaze on the contrasting embroidery on our cream lounge curtains; his days-old eyes found this detail captivating. Both my children, from birth, were extremely aware of noises, turning their heads at every distant baby cry or adult voice. As their interest in the world around them developed, it was wonderful to see them suddenly stare out of the window, amazed by their first sight of waving branches or falling snow.

As you see the natural world from a fresh perspective, experiencing it alongside your baby, reflect on the wonders of God's creation. Take time to look for a moment at the little things that bring such joy—the changing seasons, falling leaves, or clouds in a blue sky. Ask God to renew your sense of awe and wonder. Read Psalm 104:5–15 (or the whole psalm if you can) and reflect on the amazing imagery, praising God for all that he has created. How often do we fail to see his majestic power in the changing seasons or appreciate the beauty and intricacies of the natural world? Caught up in the concerns and responsibilities of adulthood, we forget to give thanks for the wonders of nature, happening all around us.

Learn from your baby! Take time to listen to the birds singing. Delight along with your child in the trees dancing merrily in the breeze, or bubbles glinting in the sunlight. Give thanks to God who created the world and praise him as you marvel anew at the work of his hands.

BIBLE VERSES
Psalm 40:5 and Psalm 104:5–15

Creator God, you made the world in all its intricate beauty, and yet I so often forget to delight in the wonders of nature. Thank you that I can see your handiwork afresh through the eyes of my child and share in a newborn's perspective on the miracles all around us. Help me to take time to recognise the way your glory and power are displayed in the changing seasons, the tiny details in a flower, or the promise of a rainbow after a storm. Thank you that when I stop concerning myself with the cares of the adult world and look with the eyes of a baby, I can feel the hope and innocent joy of appreciating small things, and give you praise. Amen

Bible index

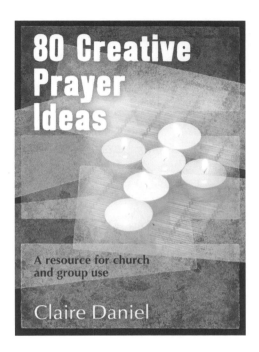

This book offers 80 imaginative and creative ideas for setting up prayer stations, practical ways of praying that involve the senses—touching, tasting, smelling, seeing and hearing, rather than simply reflecting—as we bring our hopes, fears, dreams and doubts to God. Developed from material tried and tested with small groups, the ideas provide activities ranging from bubble prayers to clay pot prayers (via just about everything else in between), and have been designed to be used with grown-ups of all ages.

80 Creative Prayer Ideas
A resource for church and group use
Claire Daniel
978 1 84101 688 7 £8.99

brfonline.org.uk

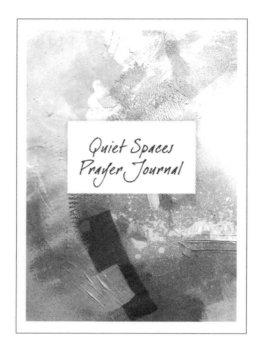

Finding God in all things, hearing God's voice for ourselves and others… the *Quiet Spaces Prayer Journal* will help you to develop and maintain a life of creative prayer. With space to write, and quotations drawn from Christian tradition and BRF's *Quiet Spaces* publication to aid reflection, this is an ideal self-purchase or gift for anyone wanting to deepen their prayer life. Each double-page spread features a quotation, allowing plenty of space to write.

Quiet Spaces Prayer Journal

978 0 85746 524 5 £9.99

brfonline.org.uk

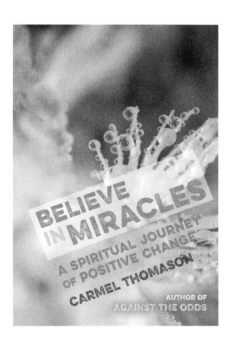

Believe in Miracles is a 40-day journey that will open your eyes to the extraordinary to be found in the everyday. Focusing on small practical steps, you are invited to follow a series of short exercises that will help bring about lasting changes in your life, leading to a more prayerful, contented and connected state of being. By setting aside as little as 20 minutes a day, you will learn to view differently your daily circumstances, your relationship with God, and your relationships with others, bringing something of the ways of heaven to earth.

Believe in Miracles
A spiritual journey of positive change
Carmel Thomason
978 0 85746 420 0 £8.99

brfonline.org.uk